Madhukar Misra

Editor

Dialysis in Older Adults

A Clinical Handbook

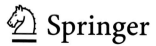 Springer

Editor
Dr. Madhukar Misra MD FRCP(UK) FACP FASN
Division of Nephrology
Department of Medicine
University of Missouri
Columbia, MO
USA

ISBN 978-1-4939-3318-1   ISBN 978-1-4939-3320-4   (eBook)
DOI 10.1007/978-1-4939-3320-4

Library of Congress Control Number: 2015959721

Springer New York Heidelberg Dordrecht London

Printed on acid-free paper

Springer Science+Business Media New York is part of Springer Science+Business Media
(www.springer.com)

Dialysis in Older Adults

The more I live, the more I learn. The more I learn, the more I realize, the less I know.
—— Michel Legrand

To
My wife Shamita, my best friend and
eternal cheerleader,
and
my children, Runjhun and Sidhant, who
mean everything to us.

Preface

I will always be indebted to three remarkable individuals who helped shape my career in ways I could never have imagined. Professor Edwina A Brown, who was a guiding force through my early days in Nephrology, Professor Karl D Nolph (deceased), who believed in me and took me under his wings within a few minutes of meeting me in Sweden and Professor Zbylut J Twardowski, a brillliant scientist and inventor, who continues to amaze me with his intellectual curiosity to this day.

Older adults comprise a steadily increasing segment of the dialysis population. They are a special patient subset with needs that are different from the average adult patient on dialysis. From the time of decision to initiate patients on dialysis, up to the time of their death or withdrawal from dialysis, nephrologists often encounter situations that may seem uniquely challenging. Their dialysis prescription as well as the management of dialysis-related complications is often based on information extrapolated from observations derived from younger adults.

This clinical handbook is not meant to provide the reader with information about the technical or other general aspects of dialysis. In fact, it assumes that one is already conversant with such information. This book attempts to embed such knowledge base with the nuances of managing an older patient with ESRD.

The authors of various chapters are recognized experts in their respective fields. This ensures clarity of content throughout the book. Each chapter ends with certain key points highlighting the main message of the chapter. This is meant to provide a quick reference tool when looking for specific information in the book.

The book is structured to provide specific topics related to dialyzing the older adult in a logical sequence. The key theme underpinning this book is the focus on managing the older patient as a whole. Consequently, the range of the book is wide and comprehensive. The early part of the book focuses on chapters related to the scope of this problem as well as the impact of pre-dialysis education on modality choice. Topics like these as well as the later topics near the end of the book deal with subjects that even though of great significance, often do not receive the attention that they deserve. The chapters related to hemodialysis focus on important issues particularly relevant to the older patient including access, hemodynamic considerations, and home hemodialysis. Likewise, the modality of peritoneal dialysis is discussed with a special emphasis on the logistical models of its delivery in various settings like home (independent and assisted) as well as nursing home.

The book is unique in several other aspects. Rather than being restricted only to chronic dialysis, it also discusses dialysis of older adults in special clinical situations like acute kidney injury and congestive heart failure. More specifically, this book's uniqueness lies in its ability to address several key areas in regard to ESRD and dialysis in the older adult patient. These include topics on blood pressure management, adequacy of dialysis, anemia, mineral bone disease, and altered pharmacology.

This book is a clinical handbook and is thus expected to serve as a quick and practical tool for easy reference when managing an older adult on dialysis. Since the content of the book builds upon the knowledge base related to dialysis, it may be useful for both the budding nephrologists and the mature physicians with specific questions.

I would like to thank all the authors for their excellent contributions and patience throughout the production of this book.

Columbia, MO, USA   Madhukar Misra

Contents

Contributors

Edwina A. Brown Imperial Renal and Transplant Centre, Hammersmith Hospital, London, UK

Aine Burns Department of Medicine, Centre for Nephrology, University College London, Royal Free NHS Foundation Trust, London, UK

Katie E. Cardone Department of Pharmacy Practice, Albany College of Pharmacy and Health Sciences, Albany, NY, USA

John T. Daugirdas Department of Nephrology, University of Illinois at Chicago, Chicago, IL, USA

Andrew Davenport UCL Center for Nephrology, University College London Medical School, Royal Free Hospital, London, UK

Robert G. Fassett School of Human Movement Studies and Nutritional Sciences, The University of Queensland, St Lucia, QLD, Australia

Darren W. Grabe Department of Pharmacy Practice, Albany College of Pharmacy and Health Sciences, Albany, NY, USA

Lina Johansson Department of Nutrition and Dietetics, Imperial College Healthcare NHS Trust, Hammersmith Hospital, London, UK

Martin K. Kuhlmann Division of Nephrology, Department of Internal Medicine, Vivantes Klinikum im Friedrichshain, Berlin, Germany

Iain C. Macdougall Department of Renal Medicine, King's College Hospital, London, UK

Renal Unit, King's College Hospital, London, UK

Madhukar Misra Division of Nephrology, Department of Medicine, University of Missouri, Columbia, MO, USA

George Sunny Pazhayattil Section of Nephrology, Yale University School of Medicine, New Haven, CT, USA

Aldo J. Peixoto Section of Nephrology, Yale University School of Medicine, New Haven, CT, USA

Paula Pond Kansas Nephrology Physicians, PA, Wichita, KS, USA

Mitchell H. Rosner Division of Nephrology, University of Virginia Health System, Charlottesville, VA, USA

Dennis L. Ross Kansas Nephrology Physicians, PA, University of Kansas School of Medicine, Wichita, KS, USA

Sergio F.F. Santos Division of Nephrology, State University of Rio de Janeiro, Rio de Janeiro, Brazil

Wendy Funk Schrag State Government Affairs, Fresenius Medical Care, Newton, KS, USA

Nicole Stankus Department of Nephrology, University of Illinois at Chicago, Chicago, IL, USA

Tushar J. Vachharajani Nephrology Section, W. G. (Bill) Hefner Veterans Affairs Medical Center, Salisbury, NC, USA

Preethi Yerram Division of Nephrology and Hypertension, Department of Internal Medicine, University of Missouri-Columbia School of Medicine, Columbia, MO, USA

Chapter 1
ESRD in the Elderly: The Scope of the Problem

Madhukar Misra

Introduction

The elderly (age >65 years) and the very elderly patients (age >75 years) constitute the fastest growing segment of patients starting dialysis. One out of every four patients starting dialysis in the USA is above the age of 75 years. There has been a huge increase in octogenarians and nonagenarians starting dialysis. Maintenance hemodialysis (HD) is often the initial dialysis modality of such patients with multiple comorbidities.

Initiating dialysis in the elderly is often fraught with multiple issues that may impact the ultimate outcome. These issues relate to awareness as well as preferences of elderly patients regarding options for renal replacement therapy (RRT), psychosocial circumstances, general frailty, comorbid load, and lack of clarity about goals of therapy (prolonging survival and/or improvement in quality of life – QOL). Palliative care and end-of-life decision making also form a major dimension of the decision-making process.

Thus, a burgeoning elderly dialysis population with its attendant comorbidities and rising costs is a major problem. This is compounded by inadequately trained nephrologists in certain basic aspects of geriatrics, making this issue even more complicated.

Dialysis decision making in the elderly is a complex process. It includes decisions involving the transition to dialysis, the pros and cons of dialysis versus no dialysis (conservative care), palliative care, as well as delineating the relative importance of survival versus quality of life (QOL). This chapter will outline the scope and magnitude of the problems faced while dialyzing the elderly population.

M. Misra, MD, FRCP (UK), FACP, FASN
Division of Nephrology, Department of Medicine,
University of Missouri, Columbia, MO, USA
e-mail: misram@health.missouri.edu

© Springer Science+Business Media New York 2016
M. Misra (ed.), *Dialysis in Older Adults: A Clinical Handbook*,
DOI 10.1007/978-1-4939-3320-4_1

1

The Steadily Rising Elderly Dialysis Population

More than 400 people per million start dialysis each year in the USA. Of these, a third (or more) are 65 years or older and account for about 42 % of costs of dialysis care in the USA. The mean age of prevalent hemodialysis patients is also on the rise worldwide. Patients above 75 years of age comprise anywhere between 18 and 40 % of prevalent patients [1]. Within the elderly population, the incident rates of dialysis initiation rise with increasing age.

The Burden of Comorbidity in the Elderly Dialysis Patient

Many elderly dialysis patients may have serious comorbidities like diabetes, heart failure, stroke, and dementia. Almost a third of them have four or more chronic conditions. The elderly dialysis patients often are frail, are prone to falls, and have impaired functional and cognitive abilities. They often suffer from a large symptom burden due to nonrenal causes. Frailty is common in dialysis patients, especially in those above 80 years. Frailty is diagnosed by the presence of three out of five qualifying symptoms (unintentional weight loss, self-reported exhaustion, slow gait speed, strength measured by a hand grip, and low physical activity) [2]. Elderly patients are more prone to falls and suffer from impaired functional and cognitive abilities. The elderly nursing home residents experience a significant loss in functional independence within the first 6 months of dialysis initiation [3]. These geriatric issues in the elderly with ESRD need special training for expert management. Geriatric nephrology is becoming an increasingly important component of dialysis practice. Given the above scenario, there has to be a paradigm shift in the way nephrologists get trained.

The Spiraling Cost of Care of the Elderly

In 2012, spending for ESRD patients increased 3.2 % to $ 28.6 billion. The steady rise in the elderly dialysis population, especially those with multiple comorbidities, contributes to the rise in the cost of dialysis care. Medicare data report even higher costs in the elderly with diabetes mellitus and congestive heart failure. Elderly patients with high scores of Charleston comorbidity index (CCI) show increased lengths of hospital stay and increased utilization of resources [4]. The higher cost of providing dialysis to the elderly (above 70) is mainly due to the actual cost of dialysis treatment rather than the cost of community and social services [5]. Dialysis provides questionable benefit in survival in the very elderly. This raises the question if the very sick elderly dialysis patients should be offered dialysis or not. This is a controversial issue and a serious discussion is out of the scope of this chapter. However, it does underscore the importance of conservative/palliative care in dialysis. It is possible that conservative and/or palliative care in certain subset of patients may be a better alternative to dialysis where not much stands to be gained in survival and/or quality of life (QOL).

The Pre-dialysis Care and Complexities of Decision Making

Limited life expectancy on dialysis together with its variable effects on the functional status and quality of life in the elderly often make it difficult to objectively assess the effect of dialysis on survival. A major problem in this area is unplanned start of dialysis. In the USA alone, 42 % of incident dialysis patients start dialysis without having seen a nephrologist. The elderly patients who start dialysis in the hospital after an acute illness face the worst outcomes, with high early and late mortality. A significant number of those who get discharged end up losing functional independence [6] affecting their QOL. The time of initiation of dialysis in debilitated nursing home elderly patients is the so-called danger period with steep decline in functional independence and a rise in the incidence of death. Timely, comprehensive, and multidisciplinary pre-dialysis care is therefore mandatory and can make transition to dialysis easier in this vulnerable population.

Modality Choice in the Elderly

Many elderly patients may not be offered a choice of dialysis modality. Almost half of the patients on HD in the BOLDE study reported that they were not offered a modality choice even though almost 80 % of the patients on HD wanted to make such a choice [7]. When deciding the modality choice in the elderly dialysis patient, a comprehensive approach should incorporate the following in regard to the patient: life expectancy, preference, and benefits versus risks of therapy.

Life Expectancy

The expected overall survival on HD versus peritoneal dialysis (PD) is similar except in the elderly >65 years of age with diabetes.

Preference

Patients may prefer PD over HD owing to greater satisfaction with care on PD, although in general, the QOL overtime between the two modalities is similar [8].

Benefits and Risks of Dialysis Modalities (HD Versus PD)

The relative benefits versus risks between PD and HD may also impact choice of modality of dialysis. The risks include modality transfer, infections, access-related issues, QOL, and satisfaction with care. In the USA, elderly patients primarily switch from PD to HD for a variety of reasons, i.e., recurrent peritonitis, failure of ultrafiltration, and catheter malfunction. Such switches increase treatment burden and cost. Infection-related morbidity is commoner in the HD patients primarily due to the preferential use of central venous catheters (CVCs) in this population. Lack of pre-dialysis care often leads to use of central venous catheters (CVCs) as the predominant mode of dialysis access. The use of CVCs is highest in North America within the developed world. Overall, PD may be associated with a lower early risk due to a reduction in infection-related morbidity (due to CVCs used in HD). However, the late risk may be higher on PD owing to switch to HD (with a CVC). There is evidence that in elderly with average or above-average life expectancy, PD confers a lower lifetime risk related for hospitalization due to sepsis compared to HD with a CVC. However, in the elderly with limited life expectancy, such rationale to prefer PD over HD (with a CVC) may not be justified.

Both home-based therapies (HD and PD) and in-center HD are options for dialysis in the elderly patients. Most elderly dialysis patients start on HD as the initial modality (in-center, satellite, or home). In general, in-center HD is the most common mode of RRT for the elderly. In the USA, in-center HD is the commonest modality [9].

Regardless of the type of dialysis, elderly patients often encounter both perceived and real challenges when considering home-based RRT. These may include concerns related to home storage space and the often required alterations for water and wiring, lack of family support, as well as physical and functional debility. Some may apprehend social isolation by the thought of home-based dialysis.

However, there is increasing interest in promoting the use of home dialysis therapies in the elderly. Besides home HD and PD, assisted PD is another form of home therapy that can be offered to the elderly. In this instance, help offered by PD nurses at patients' homes can help reduce therapy cost. Both HD and PD can be offered at nursing homes but require dedicated staff and consistent supervision by skilled off-site nephrologists.

The concept of "conservative" or non-dialysis care is gaining increasing acceptance as an alternative means to the management of elderly patients with end-stage renal disease. With properly timed multidisciplinary planning, conservative care offers a structured way for managing symptom burden and QOL in selected elderly patients

Survival of the Elderly on Dialysis

The elderly patients are a truly heterogeneous lot. In the USA, the median survival after start of dialysis falls with increasing age and is reported to be as low as 15.6 months in those above 80 [10]. In a UK study, the median survival of octogenarians was reported to be 28.9 months and was considerably higher than 8.9 months in those who chose conservative care. Such data seem to suggest that there may be some gain in survival with dialysis in this age group [11]. Of note, there has been no change in the exceptionally high one-year mortality in octogenarians and nonagenarians over the years. In this age group, the relatively flat rate of survival over the years raises the question if dialysis prolongs survival. The years spent on dialysis may be considered as a proxy for years of life gained since otherwise the patients would have died [12]. In the North Thames Dialysis Study (NDTS) [12], mortality was associated with both age and peripheral vascular disease. Thus, both age and comorbidity are important in the elderly when examining survival.

The survival on those between 70 and 80 years of age is only marginally better [13]. In the USA, the one-year survival in those 75 years or older is 54 %. Although registry data report higher mortality rates in the North American continent, one has to bear in mind that different population subgroups with differing comorbidities and access to care may impact such observations. On the other hand, relatively healthy elderly patients may do well on dialysis. Interestingly, withdrawal from dialysis is the second most common cause of cause of death in the dialysis patients above 75 years of age.

The number of comorbid conditions increases with age. As compared to an average of 2.5 chronic comorbidities afflicting individuals below the age of 70, those above 70 years of age have double the number of comorbidities. The relative risk of mortality with ESRD (as compared to individuals with no ESRD) is higher, 20, at age 45 than at the age of 75 when it is less than 3. Some studies have reported that it is not only the type but the number of comorbidities that may be important in individual patients when estimating the benefits of dialysis.

One has to bear in mind that the definition of survival may vary with the time of onset of ESRD which may be measured from the time GFR falls to less than 15 ml/min to when patients start dialysis. Other factors like late referral bias, as well as lack of meaningful data on the elderly who undergo conservative care, make survival data difficult to interpret. Time to referral and pre-dialysis planning can also impact survival in the elderly population. These patients are often referred late to the nephrologists. Available reports suggest an association between late referral and poorer outcomes (early death, prolonged and recurrent hospitalizations, etc.). Late referral may be associated with similar risk both in the elderly and the nonelderly patients. However, since relatively more elderly patients are referred late, this accounts for a large proportion of excess mortality on dialysis [14]. A recent report suggested that despite earlier referral to nephrologists, there has not been a meaningful impact on survival of elderly patients [15]. However, this report did not address issues like severity of CKD and comorbid load at the time of nephrology referral. Neither did it assess other important outcomes like hospitalization rates, cost of care, etc.

There is no doubt that multiple comorbidities and poor functional status at the start of dialysis have an adverse impact on outcome with almost 25 % mortality rate in the first 3 months. In high-risk patients with significant morbidity and functional dependence, there may not be much gain in survival. In this regard, the nursing home population is especially at risk with less than half of this population surviving after the first 9 months [3]. Multiple tools are available to help define prognosis of such patients. These take into account factors like comorbidity and mental and functional disability. These factors are then used to assign risk scores for predicting survival [16, 17]. A patient's own nephrologist may in some instances be able to provide a unique perspective on the patient's prognosis [18].

Quality of Life (QOL)

In many elderly patients on dialysis, QOL may be equally important to survival. In some, it may score even higher on the priority scale. In other words, dialysis should not only add "years to life" but should also add "life to years." For some, a visit to the HD unit may provide a means for social interaction and add to the overall quality of life. The elderly HD patients may in fact fare better than their younger counterparts on SF-36 scores [19]. In the NTDS [5], the elderly dialysis patients reported mental QOL scores that were similar to the general elderly population in the USA or the UK. However, the physical scores were lower in the dialysis patients. Data from the BOLDE study [7] show that there is no significant difference in QOL between HD and PD. However, the elderly reported less illness intrusion by PD than HD. A recent study has reported that the nephrologists would avoid dialysis recommendation if it was expected to considerably reduce QOL [20]. It is obvious that apart from patient preference, comorbidity, cognitive ability, and QOL are obvious factors that should guide dialysis decision making in the elderly patients.

Conservative Care

The concept that dialysis may not be the only option for the elderly with ESRD has gained ground over the last several years. It is now accepted that a subset of elderly ESRD patients (those with multiple comorbidities, patients who have made an informed choice, etc.) may elect to forgo dialysis and instead opt for conservative care. Conservative care is often misconstrued as palliative care. In reality it is an actively managed care of the elderly ESRD patient with emphasis on close monitoring as well as management of various clinical, psychological, and functional parameters on a regular basis. However, nephrologists' perspective on offering such care varies widely in reported studies [21]. Such disparity of perspective also exists between primary care physicians and nephrologists [22]. One of the key factors in considering such option is adopting a shared decision-making approach involving all personnel (primary physician, nephrologist, social worker, dietician, home nurse, etc.). The overall survival of patients with conservative care may be lower than those who choose to dialyze. However, such patients often end up spending a majority of their final days in the dialysis units and/or in the hospital [21].

Key Points
1. More and more elderly patients with ESRD are going on dialysis.
2. Elderly ESRD patients have multiple comorbidities and require special care owing to complex problems associated with old age.
3. This special subset of ESRD patients will need nephrologists with special skill sets particular to geriatric care.
4. The decision to choose dialysis and the type of dialysis needs a structured approach between the patients, their caregivers, the nephrologist, and other members of the multidisciplinary care team.
5. Both survival on dialysis and quality of life should be considered carefully when individual dialysis decisions are being made.
6. Conservative care on dialysis is often not discussed with the elderly patients and may be the right option for a selected group of elderly patients.

References

1. Canaud B, Tong L, Tentori F et al (2011) Clinical practices and outcomes in elderly hemodialysis patients: results from the Dialysis Outcomes and Practice Patterns Study (DOPPS). Clin J Am Soc Nephrol 6(7):1651–1662
2. Fried LP, Tangen CM, Walston J et al (2001) Frailty in older adults: evidence for a phenotype. J Gerontol A Biol Sci Med Sci 56:M146–M156
3. Kurella Tamura M, Covinsky KE, Chertow GM et al (2009) Functional status of elderly adults before and after initiation of dialysis. N Engl J Med 361:1539–1547
4. Lin Y-T, Wu P-H, Kuo M-C et al (2013) High cost and low survival rate in high comorbidity incident elderly hemodialysis patients. PLoS One 8(9), e75318
5. Grun RP, Constantinovici N, Normand C, et al for the North Thames Dialysis Study (NTDS) Group (2003) Costs of dialysis for elderly people in the UK. Nephrol Dial Transplant 18:2122–2127
6. Bjorg Thorsteinsdottir, Keith M Swetz, Jon C Tilburt. Dialysis in the Frail Elderly- a Current Ethical Problem, an Impending Ethical Crisis. J Gen Intern Med. 2013;28(11):1511–1516
7. Brown EA, Johansson L, Farrington K et al (2010) Broadening Options for Long-term Dialysis in the Elderly (BOLDE): differences in quality of life on peritoneal dialysis compared to haemodialysis for older patients. Nephrol Dial Transplant 25(11):3755–3763
8. Tamura MK, Tan JC, O'Hare AM (2012) Optimizing renal replacement therapy in older adults: a framework for making individualized decisions. Kidney Int 82:261–269
9. Brown EA, Johansson L (2011) Dialysis options for end stage renal disease in older people. Nephron Clin Pract 119(S1):c10–c13
10. U.S. Renal Data System, USRDS 2009 Annual Data Report: Atlas of Chronic Kidney Disease and End-Stage Renal Disease in the United States, National Institutes of Health, National Institute of Diabetes and Digestive and Kidney Diseases, Bethesda, MD, 2009.
11. Joly D, Anglicheau D, Alberti C et al (2003) Octogenarians reaching end-stage renal disease: cohort study of decision-making and clinical outcomes. J Am Soc Nephrol 14:1012–1102
12. Lamping D, Constantinovici N, Roderick P et al (2000) Clinical outcomes, quality of life, and costs in the North Thames Dialysis Study of elderly people on dialysis: a prospective cohort study. Lancet 356:1543–1550
13. Kooman JP, Cornelis T, van der Sande FM et al (2012) Renal replacement therapy in geriatric end stage renal disease patients: a clinical approach. Blood Purif 33(1–3):171–176

14. Schwenger V, Morath C, Hofmann A et al (2006) Late referral – a major cause of poor outcome in the very elderly dialysis patient. Nephrol Dial Transplant 21:962–967
15. Winkelmayer WC, Liu J, Chertow GM et al (2011) Predialysis nephrology care of older patients approaching end-stage renal disease. Arch Intern Med 171(15):1371–1378
16. Couchoud C, Labeeuw M, Moranne O et al (2009) A clinical score to predict 6 month prognosis in elderly patients starting dialysis for end-stage renal disease. Nephrol Dial Transplant 24:1553–1561
17. Schmidt RJ (2012) Informing our elders about dialysis: is an age-attuned approach warranted? Clin J Am Soc Nephrol 7(1):185–189
18. Moss AH, Ganjoo J, Sharma S et al (2008) Utility of the 'surprise' question to identify dialysis patients with high mortality. Clin J Am Soc Nephrol 3:1379–1384
19. Rebollo P, Ortega F, Baltar JM et al (2001) Is the loss of health-related quality of life during renal replacement therapy lower in elderly patients than in younger patients? Nephrol Dial Transplant 16:1675–1680
20. Foote C, Morton RL, Jardine M et al (2014) COnsiderations of Nephrologists when SuggestIng Dialysis in Elderly patients with Renal failure (CONSIDER): a discrete choice experiment. Nephrol Dial Transplant 29(12):2302–2309
21. Carson RC, Juszczak M, Davenport A et al (2009) Is maximum conservative management an equivalent treatment option to dialysis for elderly patients with significant comorbid disease? Clin J Am Soc Nephrol 4(10):1611–1619
22. Visser A, Dijkstra GJ, Huisman RM et al (2007) Differences between physicians in the likelihood of referral and acceptance of elderly patients for dialysis-influence of age and comorbidity. Nephrol Dial Transplant 22(11):3255–3261

Chapter 2
How to Choose the Type of Dialysis in the Elderly Patient

Lina Johansson and Edwina A. Brown

Introduction

Only a few patients over the age of 70 will be eligible for transplantation, so the older patient starting dialysis will remain on this treatment for the rest of their life. Choice of dialysis modality will not affect patient survival but will have a major impact on patient lifestyle and therefore quality of life. The decision about dialysis modality is therefore a crucially important one, and the choice should be made with the patient. This requires the clinician (nephrologist, dialysis educator, etc.) to have a realistic understanding about life on haemodialysis (HD) and peritoneal dialysis (PD) for older people in general and for the patient in particular. The patient (and family/carers) also needs appropriate unbiased education about the pros and cons of HD and PD and how both will affect their lifestyle and overall prognosis. This process is called "shared decision making". To ensure that this happens with each patient about to start dialysis, it is useful to break the process down into a series of steps as shown in Table 2.1.

L. Johansson
Department of Nutrition and Dietetics, Imperial College Healthcare NHS Trust, Hammersmith Hospital, Du Cane Road, London W12 0HS, UK

E.A. Brown, MD (✉)
Imperial Renal and Transplant Centre, Hammersmith Hospital,
Du Cane Road, London W12 0HS, UK
e-mail: e.a.brown@imperial.ac.uk

© Springer Science+Business Media New York 2016
M. Misra (ed.), *Dialysis in Older Adults: A Clinical Handbook*,
DOI 10.1007/978-1-4939-3320-4_2

Table 2.1 Steps required for choice of dialysis modality

Clinician:
Knowledge of patient's current lifestyle and need for social support
Knowledge of patient's comorbidities and how they will affect overall prognosis
Consideration of how patient will cope with HD, associated transport and vascular access
Consideration of how patient will cope with PD and whether any barriers could be overcome with assistance from family or healthcare professional
Patient:
Received and understood information about dialysis options
Considered what is important to him/her about their lifestyle and future goals
Understands how HD will affect lifestyle and goals
Understands how PD will affect lifestyle and goals
Patient and clinician together:
Determine whether patient is ready to make decision
Consider using decision aid
Patient makes decision about dialysis modality; clinician checks that patient understands implications

Features of Ageing

Most of the features of ageing are more common in patients with CKD, and in particular those approaching dialysis, than in the general population. This is partly due to the associated comorbidities and partly due to factors associated with poor kidney function. All are going to impact on the patient's lifestyle and their ability to cope with dialysis [1]. When assessing elderly patients for dialysis, the full impact of dialysis should be discussed in a realistic manner so that measures can be taken to limit further deterioration and to ameliorate the situation with appropriate multidisciplinary support.

It is helpful to divide the limitations associated with ageing into physical and psychosocial factors:

Physical: impaired physical function, falls, impaired cognitive function, poor nutritional status, arthritis, impaired vision, impaired hearing
Psychosocial: social isolation, bereavement, depression, financial problems

Impaired physical function and cognitive function are particularly common and have major implications for starting dialysis so will now be considered in more depth.

Impaired Physical Function

More frequently impaired in patients with ESRD than in the general population.

Causes

• Physical inactivity related to comorbidities and poor general well-being.

- Polypharmacy – many medications cause lethargy, postural hypotension and dizziness.
- Poor nutritional status – due to several reasons, e.g. increasing difficulties in food preparation, declining sense of taste and smell, poor dentition.
- Metabolic, e.g. acidosis, electrolyte abnormalities, hyperparathyroidism associated with renal impairment affecting muscle metabolism.
- Vicious cycle with depression – depression causing physical inactivity which then results in worsening physical function.

Assessment

- Basic activities of daily living – does the patient dress, bathe, eat independently or require assistance?
- How far can the patient walk and do they need aids – and, if so, what?
- Instrumental activities of daily living – does the patient do household tasks such as cleaning, shopping and cooking independently or require assistance?

Implications for Starting Dialysis

- Haemodialysis: consider impact of requiring transport to and from dialysis centre – time of journey, waiting at home or in dialysis centre, discomfort.
- Peritoneal dialysis: difficulty in emptying and lifting bags of dialysate; may need assistance from family or healthcare worker.
- Good evidence of often dramatic decline in physical function in the first 6 months of starting dialysis [2, 3].

Management

- Maximise treatment of underlying metabolic problems – anaemia, bone disease, acidosis and nutrition.
- Consider and treat possible depression.
- Encourage physical activity and consider referral to physiotherapy.
- Ensure that the patient has appropriate social support.

Cognitive Impairment

There is good evidence that not only is cognitive impairment more common but also that rate of decline is more rapid as kidney function declines [4, 5]. Executive function appears to be affected more than memory. The diagnosis is often not considered and only becomes apparent when difficulties are encountered when training the patient for peritoneal dialysis.

Causes

- Cerebrovascular disease associated with increased vascular risk factors in kidney disease, particularly diabetes and hypertension.
- Polypharmacy causing hypotension, confusion, drowsiness.
- Metabolic factors associated with renal disease and accumulation of "uremic toxins".

Assessment

- Ask patient and family about memory problems and whether any difficulties with daily tasks and how these have changed over time.
- Cognitive function testing is not but should become part of the routine assessment of patients with kidney disease (no different than measuring haemoglobin or plasma phosphate levels).
- Initial screen – use simple tests that can be done quickly – and remember to assess memory and executive function. Suggested simple tests are the abbreviated mental test score (AMTS), memory; 6-item cognitive impairment test (6 CIT), memory; clock drawing (CLOX 1), executive function; and Montreal Cognitive Assessment (MOCA), cognitive impairment.

Implications for Starting Dialysis

- High risk of further decline, though this needs further study.
- Haemodialysis: drops in blood pressure during dialysis could exacerbate rate of decline; visits to dialysis unit could be disorientating causing worsening confusion in patients with more advanced cognitive problems.
- Peritoneal dialysis: theoretically rate of decline could be slower than HD as blood pressure is more stable – but there are no comparative studies. However, cognitive dysfunction, particularly impaired executive function, will impede patient learning PD technique, so assistance from family or healthcare professional may be needed.

Management

- No good studies in patients with kidney disease and no evidence of benefit of drugs.
- Ensure that patient has appropriate social support.
- Assess for and treat any underlying depression.
- Avoid factors that could predispose to development of delirium when patient admitted to hospital.
- Determine wishes of patient and family about level of care if cognitive function deteriorates and patient no longer able to self-care or has capacity to make own decisions.

Haemodialysis or Peritoneal Dialysis?

Discussions relating to choice of dialysis modality should be based on the patient perspective and not on what is convenient for the doctor or biased by local politics. Patients are going to want to know whether there is any difference in survival, complications and impact on lifestyle.

Survival

There are no randomised studies comparing outcomes on HD and PD. In most countries, HD and PD populations are very different with PD mostly being used for younger patients with less comorbidity and with a higher proportion at work. This is not true, though, in France where assisted PD is widely available (see Chap. 6) and the PD population is predominantly elderly [6]. Comparisons of survival are therefore difficult and depend on multiple statistical adjustments. Modality did not affect survival of 14,512 older Canadian patients between 1990 and 1999 when adjusting for several characteristics, e.g. gender and comorbid conditions [7]. European data suggests a survival advantage for PD for patients age >70 years with a hazard ratio of 0.87 [8]. In effect, for the individual, this is small so, realistically, one should inform patients that survival is not affected by dialysis modality. The choice of HD or PD, therefore, should depend on the effect on patient lifestyle and quality of life.

Lifestyle

Both types of dialysis modality have advantages and disadvantages as shown in Table 2.2. It is important to be realistic about these to enable the patient to make the best decision for him/herself.

Table 2.2 Comparison of HD and PD from the patient perspective

Haemodialysis	Peritoneal dialysis
Hospital-based treatment	Home-based treatment
Not dependent on patient ability	Patient independence
Can provide social structure for frail elderly	Fits in with family responsibilities and social activities
Transport (journey and waiting time) needs to be added into treatment time	Can be done by carer (paid assistant or family)
Often feel washed out for hours after HD session	Less visits to hospital
Interferes with social and family life	Flexibility of manual exchanges (3–4/day) or automated cycling machine over night
Increased hospitalisation for vascular access problems	Requires space in the home to store boxes of fluid
Difficult to travel for holidays or visiting family	Treatment burden related to daily and repetitive nature of performing exchanges
	Easier to travel to go on holiday or visit family nationally or overseas

Quality of Life

There are only two studies comparing quality of life on HD and PD in older patients. The North Thames Dialysis Study was carried out in the late 1990s when 40 % of patients were on PD in the UK (most of these patients would not be offered PD today). This study showed that survival and quality of life of patients $\geq$70 years old starting dialysis were not different for HD and PD [9, 10]. BOLDE (Broadening Options for Long-term Dialysis in the Elderly) is a more recent study which has also shown that quality of life is the same on PD and HD but that there is significantly less illness and treatment intrusion for patients on PD compared to those on HD [11]. This is important information to give patients when deciding about dialysis modality.

Education in the Elderly

Education for the elderly needs to be tailored to the specific needs of this patient group. The various aspects that should be considered in any educational program for older people are listed in Table 2.3 and will be discussed in further detail below. In addition, any educational programme should involve the patient's close persons,

Table 2.3 Educational considerations and suggested actions in older people who are approaching end-stage renal disease

Educational considerations	Suggested actions
Cognitive dysfunction	May require repeating information to assist those with memory problems
	Provide information (written and verbal) that is easy to understand and avoid medical terminology jargon. Aim for a Flesch readability score of no more than 60–70 [15] by using everyday language
	Be direct and specific with the information provided
	Make information brief with 3–5 key points per section
	Use the active voice
	Use pictures to help explain information but avoid complex diagrams
Visual and hearing impairments	Use type size of at least 12 points. Use 14 points for smaller fonts such as Times New Roman. Use even larger sizes for titles
	Use serif typefaces, e.g. Times New Roman
	Use double space text where possible
	Align text to the left margin
	Ensure audio is clear and sufficiently loud enough
Physical impairments hindering attending educational sessions	Ensure the patient is able to physically attend and access the educational sessions
Less usage of Web-based educational materials	Ensure paper formats available for all information provided to the patient or offer assisted learning and devices for Internet-based learning

e.g. family, friends and caregivers, as each dialysis modality is likely to have an impact on the patients' wider support network.

Cognitive Dysfunction

The prevalence of cognitive dysfunction in older people with CKD is higher when compared to the general population. In older people living in the community or institutions in Canada, prevalence of cognitive dysfunction ranged from 11 to 30 % in those aged 65 years to >85 years [12]. By comparison, estimates of cognitive dysfunction in older people on HD can be as high as 87 % [13]. To support older people in understanding modality education, information must be accessible and easy to understand. This is not always observed as 71 % of information leaflets provided to patients about dialysis treatment options in the UK required at least the level of reading and understanding equivalent to that required for a life insurance policy [14].

Visual and Hearing Impairments

Approximately 30 % of older adults (general population in Sweden) aged 70 years have problems with their vision or hearing [16]. In unpublished data on 65 older patients who had recently started HD, 40 % had self-reported problems with their eyesight and 26 % had problems with their hearing. Therefore, several tips are provided on how to improve readability of learning materials (Table 2.3).

Physical Impairments

This has been described in detail above. It is important to ensure that educational sessions are physically accessible to older people and that transport is available where required.

Less Usage of Web-Based Educational Materials

Even though older people (aged 65 years and older) are increasingly using the Internet, only 40 % used it for internet purchases compared to 70 % of people aged 55–64 years in the UK in 2012 [17]. Therefore, educational materials need to be available in formats other than on the Internet for older people.

Education and Dialysis Modality Decision Making

It has been shown that when increasing the complexity of a task, comprehension and consistency in making decisions were poorer in older compared to younger people [18]. Therefore, systematic decision making can be more challenging for older people as it requires more effort in acquiring new information to make an informed decision. However, relying to a greater extent on simpler and less cognitively demanding strategies does not necessarily compromise the quality of decisions relative to younger people, when full, understandable information is provided (see the actions listed in Table 2.3 which can support the older person achieve greater understanding of the complex information relating to dialysis modality choices). This is because older people employ a greater use of affective decision making which makes use of gut instinct, life experience and knowledge to support the decisional process. When delivering dialysis modality education, providing real examples that contain relatable stories may help patients or readers apply the information to their personal experiences and life.

There are several other factors that can play a significant role on the dialysis modality decision-making process. Fundamentally, patients still perceive a lack of opportunity in deciding about the choice of dialysis modality. Patients also need to accept their diagnosis of end-stage renal disease and understand how their condition may progress. This can be challenging due to the absence of overt symptoms and due to the terminology used by healthcare professionals, e.g. creatinine levels. Older people also experience difficulties in understanding how dialysis would impact on their lives. This can partially be explained by the difficulties experienced by nephrologists in explaining the condition and its complexity. In addition, modality decisions can be influenced by other patients who provide a method of conceptualizing treatment impact on life. Decisions can also be influenced by the hospital environment as the frequency of exposure to HD may cause this treatment to be perceived to be of higher value or more routine compared to the less exposed home dialysis treatments of PD or home HD. Timing of information provision should ideally occur when the patient is not yet symptomatic or cognitively impaired as a result of severely reduced renal function. If a patient has already started on HD or PD acutely or has had preemptive access formed, changing to another mode of dialysis is viewed by patients as a risk and is commonly avoided.

Dialysis Modality Decision Aids

Decision aids are tools that are appropriate for use when healthcare decisions involve the weighing of benefit and harm to an individual, as well as scientific uncertainty. A recent Cochrane review found that decision aids performed well when compared to usual care interventions [19]. Decision aids, which included explicitly exploring the patient's values in relation to the pros and cons of treatment and scientific uncertainties, were successful at increasing knowledge, improving risk perceptions and reducing decisional conflict related to feeling uninformed and unclear about personal values. Decision aids also were found to reduce the number of people who were not involved in decisions and the number of people who were undecided after the intervention. They also appeared to have a positive effect on communication between the patient and the practitioner. Currently within the UK, dialysis modality decision aids have been developed for use with patients with advanced renal disease.

Audit Measures

Ascertaining whether patients are provided with the appropriate tools that enable the selection of the most appropriate form of dialysis for them should be a fundamental auditable prerequisite to assessing the success of any dialysis modality educational programme. Table 2.4 provides a list of potential audit standards.

Table 2.4 Audit standards to assess the efficacy of a dialysis modality educational programme

Area to audit	Items to audit	Potential audit measures
Patient education	Supply of both written and audio materials to support education about HD and PD Access to educational programmes Patient acquired knowledge and understanding of the different dialysis modalities Access to patient stories and environmental clues	Ensure 100 % of written or transcripts from audio materials Have a Flesch reading score between 60 and 70 Audit whether 100 % of older patients and their close persons have access to dialysis modality educational programmes Audit level of knowledge and understanding of how certain dialysis characteristics may affect lifestyle, e.g. how will HD affect ability to undertake spontaneous travel Audit whether patients are receiving balanced exposure HD and PD from patient stories and environment
Stage of dialysis decision making	Ascertaining how prepared patients are for choosing a dialysis modality immediately prior to modality selection	Stage of decision-making tool [20]
Reasoning for dialysis modality selection	Patients who have been educated appropriately will be able to state whether they have had a choice of modality and what factors contributed to their modality selection	Audit if patients perceive having had a choice of dialysis modality Audit patients' reasoning for modality selection

Key Points
1. Choice of dialysis modality will have major impact on patient lifestyle and therefore quality of life.
2. Shared decision making between patient/family and clinician enables choice of dialysis modality best suited to medical needs and lifestyle of patient.
3. Impaired physical and cognitive functions are common and have major implications for decision making and outcomes on dialysis.
4. Education and giving information need to be tailored to the needs of older patients.

References

1. Brown EA, Johansson L (2011) Epidemiology and management of end-stage renal disease in the elderly. Nat Rev Nephrol 7:591–598
2. Jassal SV, Chiu E, Hladunewich M (2009) Loss of independence in patients starting dialysis at 80 years of age or older. N Engl J Med 361:1612–1613
3. Kurella Tamura M, Covinsky KE, Chertow GM, Yaffe K, Landefeld CS, McCulloch CE (2009) Functional status of elderly adults before and after initiation of dialysis. N Engl J Med 361:1539–1547
4. Etgen T, Chonchol M, Förstl H, Sander D (2012) Chronic kidney disease and cognitive impairment: a systematic review and meta-analysis. Am J Nephrol 35:474–482
5. Buchman AS, Tanne D, Boyle PA, Shah RC, Leurgans SE, Bennett DA (2009) Kidney function is associated with the rate of cognitive decline in the elderly. Neurology 73:920–927
6. French registry for peritoneal dialysis and home haemodialysis. http://www.rdplf.org/profils/808-profil2014.html accessed 30 Sept 2015 (in French)
7. Jassal SV, Trpeski L, Zhu N, Fenton S, Hemmelgarn B (2007) Changes in survival among elderly patients initiating dialysis from 1990 to 1999. Can Med Assoc J 177:1033–1038
8. van de Luijtgaarden M, Noordzij M, Stel VS, Ravani P, Jarraya F, Collart F, Schön S, Leivestad T, Puttinger H, Wanner C, Jager KJ (2011) Effects of comorbid and demographic factors on dialysis modality choice and related patient survival in Europe. Nephrol Dial Transplant 26:2940–2947
9. Lamping DL, Constantinovici N, Roderick P, Normand C, Henderson L, Harris S, Brown E, Gruen R, Victor C (2000) Clinical outcomes, quality of life, and costs in the North Thames Dialysis Study of elderly people on dialysis: a prospective cohort study. Lancet 356:1543–1550
10. Harris SA, Lamping DL, Brown EA, Constantinovici N (2002) Clinical outcomes and quality of life in elderly patients on peritoneal dialysis versus hemodialysis. Perit Dial Int 22:463–470
11. Brown EA, Johansson L, Farrington K, Gallagher H, Sensky T, Gordon F, da Silva-Gane M, Beckett N, Hickson M (2010) Broadening Options for Long-term Dialysis for the Elderly (BOLDE): differences in quality of life on peritoneal dialysis compared to haemodialysis for older patients. Nephrol Dial Transplant 25:3755–3763
12. Graham JE, Rockwood K, Beattie BL, Eastwood R, Gauthier S, Tuokko H, McDowell I (1997) Prevalence and severity of cognitive impairment with and without dementia in an elderly population. Lancet 9068:1793–1796

13. Murray AM, Tupper DE, Knopman DS, Gilbertson DT, Pederson SL, Li S, Smith GE, Hochhalter AK, Collins AJ, Kane RL (2006) Cognitive impairment in hemodialysis patients is common. Neurology 2:216–223
14. Winterbottom A, Conner M, Mooney A, Bekker HL (2007) Evaluating the quality of patient leaflets about renal replacement therapy across UK renal units. Nephrol Dial Transplant 22:2291–2296
15. Flesch R (1946) A new readability yardstick. J Appl Psychol 32:221–233
16. Bergman B, Rosenhall U (2001) Vision and hearing in old age. Scand Audiol 30:255–263
17. Statistical Bulletin - Office for National Statistics (2014) Internet access- households and individuals. www.ons.gov.uk/ons/dcp171778_373584.pdf
18. Finucane ML, Mertz CK, Slovic P, Schmidt ES (2005) Task complexity and older adults' decision-making competence. Psychol Aging 20(1):71–84
19. Stacey D, Bennett CL, Barry MJ, Col NF, Eden KB, Holmes-Rovner M, Llewellyn-Thomas H, Lyddiatt A, Légaré F, Thomson R (2011) Decision aids for people facing health treatment or screening decisions. Cochrane Database Syst Rev (10):CD001431. doi:10.1002/14651858. CD001431.pub3
20. O'Connor AM. User manual – stage of decision making (document on internet). Ottawa: Ottawa Hospital Research Institute; © 2000. Available from http://decisionaid.ohri.ca/docs/develop/User_Manuals/UM_Stage_Decision_Making.pdf

Chapter 3
Hemodynamic Considerations During Hemodialysis in the Elderly

Madhukar Misra

Introduction

Elderly patients are prone to all the complications that can occur in a younger patient on hemodialysis (HD). However, certain complications can be particularly detrimental in this age group. The altered physiology secondary to aging as well as HD procedure itself may contribute to such complications which primarily involve cardiovascular and cerebrovascular systems.

Cardiovascular Complications

Dysautonomia is common in otherwise healthy elderly people [1]. Both sympathetic and parasympathetic nervous systems may be affected. Chronic kidney disease (CKD) also adversely impacts the autonomic nervous system. The prevalence of dysautonomia in dialysis patients has been reported to be around 41.5 % [2]. Interestingly, although the older dialysis patients have the highest prevalence of dysautonomia, coexistent chronic kidney disease does not have an augmenting effect on autonomic dysfunction. Presence of dysautonomia hampers reflex adaptive cardiovascular responses required in face of hypovolemia and/or hypotension.

In the elderly, the aging of the cardiovascular (CV) system induces multiple changes that may make such patients more prone to complications on HD (Table 3.1).

The left ventricular (LV) mass remains either unchanged or may increase with aging. Infiltration by collagen and calcium deposition into the myocardium may lead to diastolic dysfunction. Valvular abnormalities like sclerosis and regurgitation are

M. Misra, MD, FRCP (UK), FACP, FASN
Division of Nephrology, Department of Medicine, University of Missouri,
Columbia, MO, USA
e-mail: misram@health.missouri.edu

© Springer Science+Business Media New York 2016
M. Misra (ed.), *Dialysis in Older Adults: A Clinical Handbook*,
DOI 10.1007/978-1-4939-3320-4_3

21

Table 3.1 Age-related changes in heart

Changes	Consequences
Decreased HR response	Sinus pause
Longer PR Interval	Heart blocks and bundle branch blocks
Increased atrial ectopy	Atrial fibrillation
Increased ventricular ectopy	Sustained ventricular tachycardia
Altered diastolic function	Impaired ejection fraction
Aortic sclerosis	Aortic stenosis and regurgitation
Annular mitral calcification	Mitral regurgitation

Adapted from Santoro and Mancini [3], with permission)

common due to aging related calcification and myxomatous degeneration. Even though the LV contractility may be normal under physiological conditions, HD-induced stress may expose the inability of the CV system to respond by mounting a suboptimal inotropic and chronotropic response [3].

The HD procedure per se is now known to induce circulatory stress in vulnerable vascular beds. Such stress in the coronary vasculature leads to diminished myocardial perfusion and stunning of the myocardium [4–7]. As a result of the abovementioned pathophysiological changes as well as HD-induced myocardial stunning, elderly patients may be prone to complications both during and in between HD. During HD, hypotension and/or chest pain (reduced coronary reserve) may become an issue. In the interdialytic period, patients may become more prone to pulmonary edema owing to diastolic dysfunction.

Intradialytic hypotension (IDH) may also be consequent to some changes that are specific to this age group. For example, hypoalbuminemia, a common finding in the elderly, predisposes to IDH by impairing vascular refilling. Besides, both myocardial ischemia and hypovolemia may contribute to IDH. Arteriolar and venoconstriction are crucial adaptive mechanisms in face of hypovolemia. Both these responses may be maladaptive in the elderly patients owing to altered arteriolar stiffness (loss of elasticity) as well as altered neurovegetative response which is common in old age. This abnormality prevents an increase in venous tone, impairing venous return, reducing cardiac filling, stroke volume, and blood pressure [8]. Dysautonomia may prevent an appropriate rise in heart rate in an underfilled ventricle during a severe hypovolemic episode during HD. This abnormality may get even worse by triggering of Bezold-Jarisch reflex and may lead to further worsening of hypotension [3].

The prevalence of hypertension, CHF, and coronary heart disease rises with age. Age-related senescence may lead to degenerative changes in the cardiac conductive system and reduce the density of pacemaker cells in the sinoatrial node. These pro-arrhythmogenic pathologies may cause both intradialytic and interdialytic arrhythmias. The incidence of arrhythmias in the dialysis population ranges anywhere between 17 and 76 % and is higher in older patients [9–12]. In addition, electrolyte disturbances like hypokalemia, consequent to malnutrition (often common in the elderly), may further predispose the elderly to arrhythmias. As reported earlier [3], the prevalence of atrial fibrillation (AF) increases with age even in the absence of clinically detectable cardiac disease. This together with the changes mentioned in Table 3.1 may make elderly patients more prone to potentially fatal rhythm disturbances like atrial fibrillation with rapid ventricular response. AF in the elderly HD patients may not only worsen the IDH but also impair diastolic filling in an already compromised heart even in the interdialytic period. The risk of cerebral embolism is likewise increased. However, recent data do not support the use of warfarin for primary prevention in HD patients with AF [13, 14].

Cerebrovascular Complications

The poor hemodynamic reserve and tolerance during HD may make other organs also prone to ischemia-related injury. The brain is especially vulnerable in this regard. Impairment of cognition and psychomotor abilities is common in elderly HD patients. The clinical picture involving cerebral circulation may be chronic or subacute in presentation.

Chronic clinical presentation may range from poor decision making and subtle memory disturbances to more serious manifestations like depression as well as multi-infarct dementia (Fig. 3.1). Both cortical and subcortical injury patterns have been described. Subcortical injury involves the watershed vascular zones of neural vasculature and is worsened by repeated hemodynamic insults. Subcortical

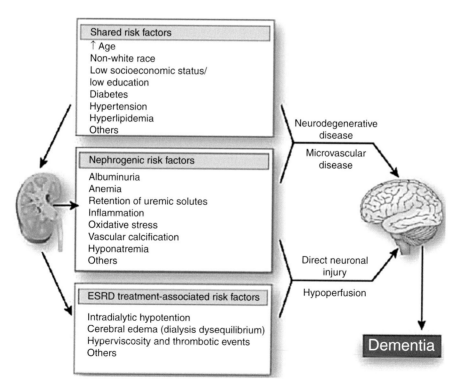

Fig. 3.1 Possible causes of dementia in the elderly (Reproduced with permission from Tamura and Yaffe [23])

Table 3.2 Neurological injury in elderly HD patients

Cause	Consequence
Altered cerebral cortical reserve	Frontal cortical atrophy (associated with dialysis vintage)
Intradialytic hypotension	Repetitive brain ischemia, atrophy
Microbubble injury	Repetitive brain ischemia
Osmotic demyelination syndrome	Neurocognitive disturbances

Adapted from Santoro and Mancini [3], with permission

functions like decision making primarily get affected [15], whereas cortical functions like memory and vocabulary are spared. Such injury may also disrupt neural connections between cortex and subcortical regions leading to mood disorders, depression, etc. This can have secondary consequences such as loss of functional independence [16, 17].

Several possible etiologies have been put forth to account for these sequelae, including cortical atrophy, water and electrolyte imbalance, repeated hemodynamic instability, etc. (Table 3.2). The frontal cortex is especially prone to ischemia-induced hypoxia [18]. The frontal atrophy seen in HD patients appears at a relatively younger age and worsens with age, presence of diabetes, and dialysis duration. Another often under recognized potential cause of chronic neuronal damage is microbubbles produced during HD. Microbubbles are very small (equal to or smaller than erythrocytes – diameter less than 10 micrometers) and may easily pass through pulmonary capillaries to the left side of the heart and onwards to the brain causing ischemic injury [19]. HD-induced recurrent hemodynamic stress has also been shown to cause progressive white matter injury of the brain [20].

The clinical presentation of subacute complication often involves the very elderly patients (above 80 years) on HD. It may range from subtle changes (aspecific behavioral disturbances and altered sensorium) to frank convulsions. It is caused by rapid reduction of plasma urea concentrations leading to intracellular shift of plasma water causing brain edema (dialysis disequilibrium syndrome – DDS). In rare cases, demyelination may be responsible. This may be asymptomatic and often reversible (mean 5 weeks) suggesting edema rather than frank myelinolysis as the likely etiology and may be diagnosed by MRI [21].

In summary, the cognitive and psychiatric manifestations in the elderly patients on HD can be due to a multitude of factors that include age-induced changes, ischemic cortical atrophy, rapid osmolar shifts, cerebral microembolism, and demyelination.

Prevention and Management of Complications

Given the above discussion, it is imperative that the HD prescription should be individualized to prevent the above complications.

Avoidance of hypotension is paramount in the elderly for the above-stated reasons. The ultrafiltration rate (UFR) is the main determinant of IDH. In the absence of UF, hypotension is generally unlikely. UFR of less than 10 ml/kg/hour may also be excessive for elderly patients, especially who are malnourished and frail with low serum albumin. The use of cooled dialysate prevents hypotensive episodes and may have a particularly beneficial role in the elderly by preventing white matter injury to the brain [20].

It is important to bear in mind that rapid reduction of blood urea levels should be avoided owing to enhanced propensity to DDS in the elderly. Thus, use of small surface area dialyzers and low blood flows, at least in the initial few HD treatments, makes clinical sense. In the same context, HD prescription should be carefully individualized to prevent hypokalemia (low dialysate potassium predisposes to cardiac arrhythmias) and hypocalcemia (higher dialysate calcium may enhance cardiac contractility). Wherever possible the dialysate sodium should be individualized and kept as close to the patient's plasma sodium as possible, and low dialysate sodium should be avoided.

Careful attention must be paid to the use of antihypertensive medications. The pharmacokinetics of various medications is altered in the elderly. IDH in this group may often be the result of lack of attention to details of prescription of antihypertensive therapy in the elderly. Besides hypotension, injudicious use of antihypertensive drug therapy may lead to fistula thrombosis in the interdialytic period, especially when patients are advised to take their antihypertensive medication/s post HD in an effort to avoid IDH. This is discussed in detail in Chap. 12.

Frequent HD (short daily and nocturnal HD) regimens may also be useful in the elderly. They may not only help lower the UFR (and thus prevent IDH episodes) but also protect against LVH, reduce incidence of hypertension and prevent rapid electrolyte shifts. The putative benefits of more frequent HD also include beneficial effects on endothelium dependent and independent vaso-reactivity, baroceptor sensitivity, and autonomic dysfunction [22] (Table 3.3).

Table 3.3 Potential benefits of Intensive HD in the elderly

Clinical problem	Pathophysiology	Potential benefits
Dialysis-related hypotension	IHD and valvular heart disease LVH and diastolic dysfunction Dysautonomia Arterial stiffness Hypoalbuminemia High UFR	↓ myocardial stunning, ↓ IHD ↓ LVH ↑ autonomic function ↑ arterial compliance ↓ malnutrition ↓ UFR
Cardiac events	IHD Dialysis-related hypotension Arrhythmias Dysautonomia Electrolyte changes	↑ endothelial function, ↓ UFR, ↓ arterial hypertension ↑ hemodynamic stability ↓ arterial hypertension, ↓ IHD, ↓ electrolyte shifts ↑ autonomic function ↑ autonomic function ↓ electrolyte shifts
Cerebral disturbances	Cerebrovascular disease Arterial hypertension Dialysis-related hypotension Dialysis disequilibrium syndrome	↑ endothelial function, ↓ arterial hypertension ↓ arterial hypertension ↑ hemodynamic stability ↓ malnutrition, slower urea clearance

Adapted from Cornelis et al. [22], with permission

Key Points
1. Elderly patients are particularly vulnerable to cardiovascular and cerebrovascular complications on HD.
2. Age-related morphological changes in the heart, brain, and blood vessels as well as impaired cardioprotective reflexes are an important cause of these complications.
3. The processes inherent to the HD procedure per se can also predispose to such complications by further stressing a compromised vascular state (ultrafiltration, clearance of antihypertensive medications on HD, osmolar shifts on HD).
4. These complications may present with a range of symptoms from mild (weakness, confusion) to serious (chest pain, seizures, etc.).
5. HD prescription in the elderly needs to be carefully individualized to prevent these complications.
6. More frequent HD regimens may have potential role in preventing these complications but are not commonly available.

References

1. Malik S, Winney RJ, Ewing DJ (1986) Chronic renal failure and the older dialysis patients only ($P<0.05$). cardiovascular autonomic function. Nephron 43:191–195
2. Jassal SV, Douglas JF, Stout RW (1998) Prevalence of central autonomic neuropathy in elderly dialysis patients. Nephrol Dial Transplant 13:1702–1708
3. Santoro A, Mancini E (2010) Hemodialysis and the elderly patient: complications and concerns. J Nephrol 23(S15):S80–S89
4. McIntyre CW (2010) Recurrent circulatory stress: the dark side of dialysis. Semin Dial 23:449–451
5. McIntyre CW (2010) Haemodialysis-induced myocardial stunning in chronic kidney disease – a new aspect of cardiovascular disease. Blood Purif 29:105–110
6. McIntyre CW, Burton JO, Selby NM, Leccisotti L, Korsheed S, Baker CS, Camici PG (2008) Hemodialysis-induced cardiac dysfunction is associated with an acute reduction in global and segmental myocardial blood flow. Clin J Am Soc Nephrol 3:19–26
7. Burton JO, Jefferies HJ, Selby NM, McIntyre CW (2009) Hemodialysis induced cardiac injury: determinants and associated outcomes. Clin J Am Soc Nephrol 4:914–920
8. Kooman JP, Gladziwa U, Bocker G, van Bortel LM, van Hooff JP, Leunissen KM (1992) Role of the venous system in hemodynamics during ultrafiltration and bicarbonate dialysis. Kidney Int 42:718–726
9. Santoro A, Mancini E, Spongano M, Rossi M, Paolini F, Zucchelli P (1990) A haemodynamic study of hypotension during hemodialysis using electrical bioimpedance cardiography. Nephrol Dial Transplant 5(Suppl 1):147–151
10. Santoro A, Mancini E, Gaggi R et al (2005) Electrophysiological response to dialysis: the role of dialysate potassium content and profiling. Contrib Nephrol 149:295–305
11. Abe S, Yoshizawa M, Nakamishi N et al (1996) Electrocardiographic abnormalities in patients receiving hemodialysis. Am Heart J 131:1137–1144
12. Rombolà G, Colussi G, De Ferrari ME, Frontini A, Minetti L (1992) Cardiac arrhythmias and electrolyte changes during haemodialysis. Nephrol Dial Transplant 7:318–322

13. Winkelmayer WC, Liu J, Setoguchi S, Choudry NK (2011) Effectiveness and safety of warfarin initiation in older hemodialysis patients with atrial fibrillation. Clin J Am Soc Nephrol 6:2662–2668
14. Chou CY et al (2010) Outcome of atrial fibrillation among patients with end-stage renal disease. Nephrol Dial Transplant 25:1225–1230
15. Pereira AA, Weiner DE, Scott T, Chandra P, Bluestein R, Griffith J, Sarnak MJ (2007) Subcortical cognitive impairment in dialysis patients. Hemodial Int 11(3):309–314
16. Lamar M, Charlton RA, Morris RG, Markus HS (2010) The impact of subcortical white matter disease on mood in euthymic older adults: a diffusion tensor imaging study. Am J Geriatr Psychiatry 18:634–642
17. Alexopoulos GS, Kiosses DN, Klimstra S, Kalayam B, Bruce ML (2002) Clinical presentation of the "depression-executive dysfunction syndrome" of late life. Am J Geriatr Psychiatry 10(1):98–106
18. Kanai H, Hirakata H, Nakane H et al (2001) Depressed cerebral oxygen metabolism in patients with chronic renal failure: a positron emission tomography study. Am J Kidney Dis 38:S129–S133
19. Polaschegg HD, Levin NW (2004) Hemodialysis machines and monitors: air embolies. In: Horl WH (ed) Replacement of renal function by dialysis. Kluwer Academic Publishers, London, pp 325–449
20. Eldehni MT, Odudu A, McIntyre CW (2015) Randomized clinical trial of dialysate cooling and effects on brain white matter. J Am Soc Nephrol 26:957–965
21. Tarhan NC, Agildere AM, Sibel Benli U, Nurhan Ozdemir F, Aytekin C, Can U (2004) Osmotic demyelination syndrome in end-stage renal disease after recent hemodialysis. AJR Am J Roentgenol 182:809–816
22. Cornelis T, Kotanko P, Goffin E, Kooman JP, van der Sande FM, Chan CT (2011) Can intensive hemodialysis prevent loss of functionality in the elderly ESRD patient? Semin Dial 24(6):645–652
23. Tamura MK, Yaffe K (2011) Dementia and cognitive impairment in ESRD: diagnostic and therapeutic strategies. Kidney Int 79:14–22

Chapter 4
The Pros and Cons of Home vs. In-Center Dialysis in the Elderly

Dennis L. Ross, Wendy Funk Schrag, and Paula Pond

Introduction

The Dialysis Population

Chronic renal failure requiring dialysis had been on the increase for several years until 2007 when the incidence of new end-stage renal disease (ESRD) patients per million population fell by 2.0 % (Fig. 4.1). The growth of patients ages 65–74, however, has increased which may be a reflection of the "baby boomers" developing renal failure (Fig. 4.2). Additionally, treatment of the elderly may be increasing due to longer life spans, a greater acceptance of dialysis as a modality to sustain life, and the availability of dialysis because of the proliferation of dialysis centers. For the first time in 2010, the number of patients doing in-center hemodialysis declined, and the number of patients that started home therapies, in particular, peritoneal dialysis, increased. For the majority of elderly patients with renal failure, the choice of therapy has been in-center dialysis with 96 % performing in-center hemodialysis, 3.5 % doing CAPD/CCPD, and only 0.3 % home hemodialysis [1].

Longevity in the general population varies significantly from country to country with Japan having the longest life span averaging 82.73 years (79.25 years for men and 86.06 years for women). Compared to Japan, the United States is ranked number 40.

D.L. Ross, MD (✉)
Kansas Nephrology Physicians, PA, Clinical Professor University
of Kansas School of Medicine, Wichita, KS, USA
e-mail: dross@kansasnephrology.com

W.F. Schrag
Vice President State Government Affairs, Fresenius Medical Care, Newton, KS, USA

P. Pond, APRN
Kansas Nephrology Physicians, PA, Clinical Professor University
of Kansas School of Medicine, Wichita, KS, USA

© Springer Science+Business Media New York 2016
M. Misra (ed.), *Dialysis in Older Adults: A Clinical Handbook*,
DOI 10.1007/978-1-4939-3320-4_4

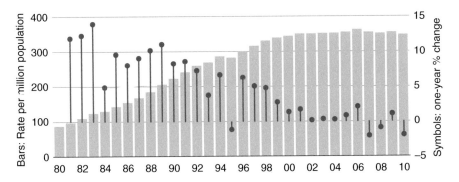

Fig. 4.1 Incidence of new ESRD patients (U.S. Renal Data System, USRDS 2011 Annual Data Report: Atlas of End-Stage Renal Disease in the United States, National Institutes of Health, National Institute of Diabetes and Digestive and Kidney Diseases, Bethesda, MD, 2011)

Fig. 4.2 Ages of new ESRD patients (U.S. Renal Data System, USRDS 2011 Annual Data Report: Atlas of End-Stage Renal Disease in the United States, National Institutes of Health, National Institute of Diabetes and Digestive and Kidney Diseases, Bethesda, MD, 2011)

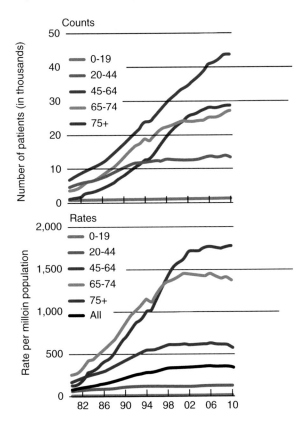

Men in the United States reach an average age of 75.25 and women 80.51 years of age with the overall average age of 75.35 years [2]. With the average lifespan of Americans being 75.35 years, it can be assumed that the elderly starting dialysis at age 70 or older would normally have only five years of survival remaining. Although the United States has a lower life expectancy than many other countries, there are a greater number of dialysis patients in the elderly group. In some countries with socialized medicine, there has been a perception of a low acceptance rate for elderly patients for dialysis. This acceptance rate has appeared to change in the UK with the advent of peritoneal dialysis, a less costly option [3]. Dialysis rationing has been described in South Africa because of too few dialysis facilities and health care workers. In the United States in the 1960s, there was a similar rationing of dialysis before Medicare and private insurance provided coverage for long-term dialysis [4]. With Medicare and privatized insurance, the United States has not placed age restrictions on dialysis so far. If the nephrologists feel the patient is able to tolerate the therapy, dialysis is an option to prolong one's life or act as a bridge until kidney function returns to baseline. Therefore, it is not uncommon to see 80- or 90-year-old patients being placed on dialysis, potentially prolonging life beyond their normal longevity.

The Move Away from Home Therapies

The first home hemodialysis in the United States was performed by Nose in 1961 [5]. With the development of the Scribner shunt, home hemodialysis began to flourish. By the 1970s, home hemodialysis accounted for as much as 40 % of all patients on dialysis. The prevalence of home hemodialysis began to fall, however, as the numbers of dialysis facilities increased and reimbursement through Medicare made payment of the treatment possible, whether at home or in-center.

Today there is considerable diversity worldwide among therapies chosen for dialysis. In New Zealand and Australia, home hemodialysis is performed on 16.3 % and 9.3 % of the ESRD population, respectively, as compared to 0–3.3 % in other countries (Fig. 4.3).

International Trends in Home Hemodialysis

There is considerable disparity in the use of home therapies for dialysis between countries. Australia and New Zealand have always had a much higher population of home patients, but in many countries, the prevalence of home hemodialysis has fallen. Remarkably, Australia and New Zealand have maintained a high number on home hemodialysis. In a review by Disney from 1995, in Australia 68 % of the patients were receiving hemodialysis and 31 % CAPD. Of the patients dialyzing at home, the majority (62 %) used CAPD, and the remainder were on home hemodialysis. In New Zealand, 44 % of the patients are on hemodialysis with 83 % dialyzing at home. The majority (65 %) use CAPD [6]. In these countries, like others, there has been a declining home hemodialysis population, but there has been a resurgence of interest driven by a variety of factors. These include the desire for cost containment and the lower mortality risk compared to in-center treatments and peritoneal dialysis.

Mcgregor, Agar, and Blagg reviewed international trends in home hemodialysis and found little correlation to other renal replacement therapies, disease states, healthcare expenditures, or population density. They did find a strong correlation

Fig. 4.3 Renal
replacement therapies
in different countries
(U.S. Renal Data System,
USRDS 2011 Annual Data
Report: Atlas of End-Stage
Renal Disease in the
United States, National
Institutes of Health,
National Institute of
Diabetes and Digestive
and Kidney Diseases,
Bethesda, MD, 2011)

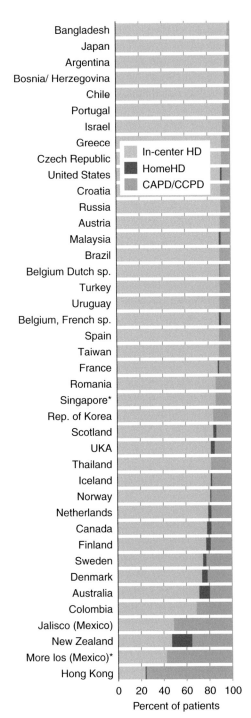

between national per capita healthcare expenditure and provision of renal replacement therapies, but no correlation with the use of home hemodialysis. Gross national income per capita also had no correlation with home hemodialysis, and there was an inverse correlation between median age and home hemodialysis [7]. In part, the resurgence of interest in home hemodialysis has been sparked by the advent of nocturnal dialysis. Performing the therapy at night gives the patient improved quality of life, more dietary and fluid freedom, need for fewer antihypertensive medications and phosphate binders, return of daytime freedom, and the capacity for full-time employment. Moreover, home hemodialysis has been found to be less expensive than in-center treatments due to the elimination of the high cost of nursing care and building costs.

Machine Options for Home Hemodialysis

There are currently two machines generally available for home hemodialysis. The Fresenius Home K is an adaption of the K in-center machine with software that helps the patient and support person doing home dialysis (Fig. 4.4).

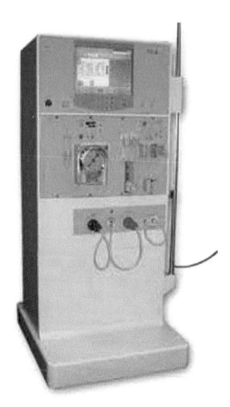

Fig. 4.4 Fresenius Home
K machine

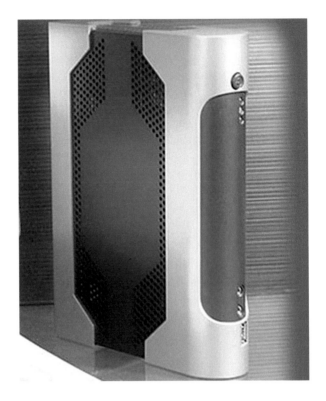

Fig. 4.5 iCare Monitoring
(http://www.fmcna.com/
fmcna/HomeTherapies/
iCareMonitoring/icare.
html)

It leads the patient and helper through the process of setting up the tubing and priming the machine. Its size is smaller than the K machine and has a connection to the Internet that can allow central monitoring from a national center. The device for central monitoring is called the *iCare Monitoring* (Fig. 4.5).

To further protect the patient, a wireless wetness detector can be placed near the needle sites, and if wetness is detected, the device will stop the blood pump (Fig. 4.6).

The Home K does require a special water system that is dependent on the quality of the patient's local water. Deionizing tanks may be required in addition to the reverse osmosis system to create quality water. Space may be a limiting factor in using a Home K machine.

The Home K machine has been used for both daytime and nocturnal dialysis. In some centers a standard K machine or other standard hemodialysis machine may be used for home therapy. These machines would not offer a step-by-step procedure on the computer screen to lead the patient through the process and would not have the Internet connection for central monitoring.

The Home K machine requires two 20 amp separate circuits. One circuit is needed for the Home K machine itself and one circuit for the reverse osmosis system. A GFI (Ground Fault Interrupter) is mandatory to prevent any circuit overload. The water does not have to meet EPA standards, and it uses cold water. The minimal standard PSI is 40 for well water.

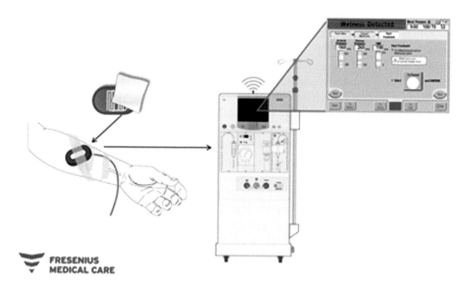

Fig. 4.6 Wireless wetness detector (http://www.fmcna.com/fmcna/HomeTherapies/home-therapies.html)

Fig. 4.7 NxStage machine
(http://www.rubindialysis.
org/homeTherapy.html)

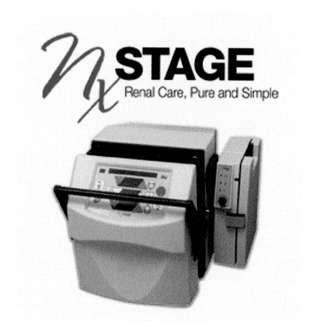

The NxStage machine was developed especially for home therapies but is also used for in-hospital CRRT (Fig. 4.7). The treatment has a unique process of treatment for uremia utilizing a slow dialysate flow rate that maximally concentrates urea and other uremic toxins in the filtrate. By using a very slow dialysate flow rate, a smaller amount of fluid is required. While being very efficient, the slow rate may not remove toxins as effectively because of the super saturation of the dialysate solution. Nevertheless, the device has rejuvenated interest in home hemodialysis because it is easier to learn with very intuitive steps to carry out the therapy.

The dialyzer and tubing are packaged as a single disposable unit making it possible to set up the machine in only 15 min. Using replacement fluid bags, the device does not require a special water system; however, the downside of using replacement bags is a higher cost per treatment as the bags are more expensive as compared to a K machine with a separate water treatment system. By using the company's Pureflow device to create sterile dialysate solution, the overall cost can be reduced.

The water must meet EPA standards to use Pureflow. In areas of the country where the nitrate and sulfate concentrations are high, Pureflow cannot be used. The water connects directly to the faucet, garden hose, washing machine, or below the sink. All of these attachments come with the NxStage kit. The blue water source line is standard and cannot be lengthened. The drain line has a maximum of 40 ft, and the electrical connection is a grounded outlet only.

There have been other machines that have come and gone over time which have been used for home hemodialysis. One example is the AKSYS home dialysis machine that was designed specifically for home hemodialysis. The system was disinfected by heat but did experience several problems with breakdowns.

More devices are being investigated for home dialysis, so we can anticipate more options in the future. It can be expected that these devices will become more automated and patient friendly and would simplify the water system. They will likely be able to transmit data to the home dialysis department allowing the treatment to be tracked by the home dialysis nurse.

Special Considerations of the Elderly

The elderly with renal failure often face a number of formidable issues in addition to their renal failure. Because vascular disease is particularly prominent prior to starting dialysis, the elderly patient may not tolerate dialysis as well. They often have underlying heart disease with reduced cardiac function. Their peripheral vasculature has significant atherosclerosis that leads to intermittent claudication, limb ulcers, and amputation. Placement of the vascular access used for hemodialysis can lead to worsening of their circulatory compromise and/or loss of a limb. They may develop "steal syndrome" and subsequent neurological damage to their hand. They also may have an increased incidence of neurological issues such as TIAs or stroke as a result of carotid artery stenosis. They usually become very weak with dialysis treatments. The 3-day period between treatments can lead to congestive heart failure and pulmonary edema because of the inability to effectively remove all of the accumulated fluid using a three-time a week treatment regimen. In addition, cardiac status may be compromised which makes it difficult to tolerate fluid build-up between treatments. Appetite is often already suppressed and may frequently worsen with dialysis leading to protein malnutrition that in turn leads to poorer outcomes.

Training for home hemodialysis involves training a "helper" to assist the patient. Usually, this is the spouse. A suitable partner is necessary for successful home treatments, and not having a partner capable of learning the treatment may be a hindrance. Additionally, there may be medical issues with the partner that compromise his/her ability to perform the treatment, or they may have disabilities limiting their own ability to provide any care. They may have poor vision, lack of dexterity or strength, and inability to learn a new technique. The housing situation may be inadequate for the storage of equipment and supplies. Fear about performing a home treatment may prevent the patient or helper from choosing this modality. The family may be concerned that it would place too much burden on the caregiver.

Financial issues may also push the patient to do in-center dialysis. Although Medicare provides nearly universal health care coverage for most individuals at the age of 65, it doesn't cover everything. The elderly often have fixed incomes that preclude them from affording expensive medications even when they have partial prescription coverage. Medicare does not cover an assistant at home to do the therapy. The increased electrical and water costs of the home therapy may be a strain on their fixed income. Transportation to and from the dialysis unit may be a problem, and the patient may not be able to drive himself to the dialysis facility and may have to rely on a family member or public transportation.

The elderly are also at increased risk for falling. Abdel-Pahman EM et.al described in a pilot study over a 1-year period a 26.3 % incidence of falls in their dialysis population [8]. The elderly, particularly females, were prone to falling. The greater the number of falls, the worse was the outcome. Due to an increased risk of bleeding because of the uremic state and anticoagulants that the patients receive, serious complications such as subdural hematomas can have disastrous results. Hip fractures resulting from falls will often lead to nursing home placement and subsequent death.

It has been well recognized that renal failure patients have an increased problem with depression, a sense of loss of control, general fatigue, and lack of energy. The elderly patients on dialysis are particularly prone to these symptoms. More frequent dialysis treatments may tend to improve these symptoms since the treatments can be gentler and less aggressive.

Benefits of Home Hemodialysis for the Elderly

While the problems that the elderly face are similar to younger patients with multiple comorbidities, they generally do not tolerate aggressive treatments as well. Therefore, slower treatments can be advantageous. The standard in-center dialysis treatment program today is of 3–4 h duration, 3 days a week. With home therapies, the longer and gentler treatments can be done in a cost-effective way. Short daytime or slower nighttime treatments can be done four to six times per week.

When Ipema et.al studied protein intakes between day and night hemodialysis patients, they found that the protein intake of patients improved significantly when they transitioned from daytime therapy to nighttime. With longer treatments, the patients' phosphate levels remained stable even though their phosphorus intake was greater [9]. These factors suggest the nutritional status of the elderly dialysis patient may be enhanced with more frequent, longer and gentler treatments. Similarly, Uldall et al. described their early experience with home nocturnal dialysis patients dialyzing five to seven nights a week. They were successful in discontinuing phosphate binders and allowing a higher phosphate diet. Their patients experienced increased energy and stamina.

Sleep disturbances are common in the elderly. Improvement of sleep apnea was seen in the Canadian experience with home nocturnal dialysis. The conversion from conventional in-center dialysis to nocturnal dialysis was associated with a reduction in the frequency of apnea and hypopnea from 25+/−25 to 8+/8− episodes per hour of sleep ($p=0.03$). The apnea-hypopnea index was greater on the nights when no dialysis was being performed as opposed to the nights of dialysis [10, 11]. The majority of patients also reported improved sleep.

The elderly have an increased risk of hypotension, cerebral and cardiac events, malnutrition, infection, sleep abnormalities, and psychological complications after initiation of dialysis. Home nocturnal hemodialysis is a less aggressive treatment and thus may be advantageous due to the comorbidities of the elderly. Such patients do particularly well with regard to these complications when doing home nocturnal hemodialysis.

Since fluid control can be problematic for the elderly, particularly for the extended 3-day periods, a nocturnal treatment program that offers at least quotidian therapy is an attractive option in controlling fluid balance. Improvement of left ventricular hypertrophy in home nocturnal dialysis patients has been established.

Therefore, taken altogether it becomes apparent that more frequent dialysis, slower dialysis, and extended treatments can potentially improve the outcomes and quality of life of the elderly patient on dialysis.

Benefits of Early Education

If the patient is seen early in their course by the nephrologist, the patient is more likely to choose a home therapy, less likely to start dialysis with a catheter and overall have better outcomes (Table 4.1).

Studies at Fresenius Medical Care have shown that a proactive educational program (Treatment Options Program or TOPS) for patients with progressive renal disease will more often lead to choosing a home therapy. Education also leads to early placement of the access so it can be functional when dialysis is needed (Fig. 4.8).

Without the physician encouraging home hemodialysis, the patient and their family will not likely choose this form of treatment since the patient turns to the physician for advice and direction as to which therapy to choose. When patients

Table 4.1 Early Education Outcomes

	None	0–12 mo.	>12 mo.
All	43.0	31.7	25.4
Mean age (yrs)	61.6	62.7	63.7
0–19	1.1	1.2	1.4
20–44	13.6	11.3	9.6
45–64	39.7	38.4	36.4
65–74	21.9	24.2	25.8
75+	23.7	24.9	26.7
Female	42.8	43.4	42.8
Race			
White	63.2	65.7	70.6
Blk.Af Am	29.6	27.6	23.3
Native American	1.2	1.4	1.1
Asian	4.9	5.2	4.9
Hispanic	17.0	13.4	11.1
Access at initiation			
Catheter	88.9	68.0	53.5
Fistula	3.2	16.9	26.3
Graft	1.2	3.4	4.0
Maturing fistula	11.3	17.9	17.1
Maturing graft	1.7	2.5	2.0
ESA use	2.0	31.5	41.8
Dietary care	0.2	14.1	17.1
eGFR			
<5	9.5	5.2	5.1
5 ≤ 10	35.4	36.4	38.4
10 ≤ 15	28.6	36.1	36.7
≥15	19.5	20.1	18.5
DM (comorbidity)	49.4	56.9	55.8
Primary diagnosis			
Diabetes	38.9	49.1	46.9
Hypertension	28.9	28.0	26.9
Glomerulonephritis	4.7	6.6	8.9
Cystic kidney	0.9	2.2	4–6

U.S. Renal Data System, USRDS 2011 Annual Data Report: Atlas of End-Stage Renal Disease in the United States, National Institutes of Health, National Institute of Diabetes and Digestive and Kidney Diseases, Bethesda, MD, 2011

were asked who first made them aware of home hemodialysis, only 35 % stated that their physician first made them aware of the home treatment. When asked who rec-ommended home hemodialysis, only 11 % of the time the recommendation was made by the physician (Fig. 4.9).

Early education will lead to more patients choosing a home therapy; therefore, it is often helpful to consider the 30/20/10 rule. At a GFR of 30 ml/min, discussions

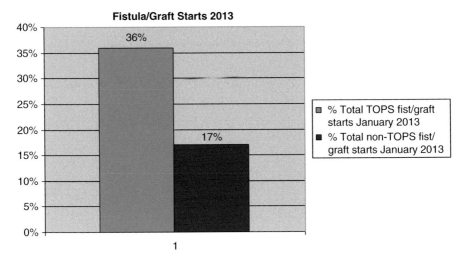

Fig. 4.8 Early placement of access in patients attending proactive education program vs those not participating. (Unpulished raw data)

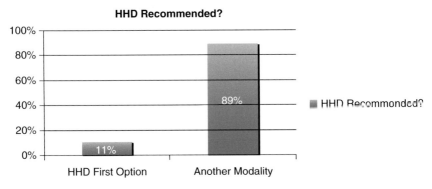

Fig. 4.9 Home hemodialysis recommended by physician (Chadwick Martin Bailey; NxStage Home Hemodialysis Patient Research, October 2008 p. 1–44)

regarding kidney failure and dialysis should be started with the patient and their family. All options should be presented, but home therapies can be encouraged if the patient is a good candidate. Since no one therapy fits every individual, it is realized that home hemodialysis is not the only option, but it is a more viable option than what is being encouraged today. At a GFR of 20 ml/min, a discussion for vascular access placement may be considered with the caveat that progression to ESRD is slower in the elderly. Usually grafts should not be placed early since the graft will have a limited lifespan and can be placed and used usually within 3–4 weeks.

At a GFR of 10 ml/min, dialysis will typically be started due to uremic symptoms. The 30/20/10 rule is helpful but should be used in the context of the rate of deterioration of renal function. There are patients whose renal function may deteriorate very slowly over time. If the rate of decline of renal function is slow, placement of an access could be delayed. To assess the rate of decline, using the reciprocal of the creatinine over time can help predict future value that in turn can assist in choosing the right time for access placement. The practitioner should keep in the mind that the muscle mass of the elderly is reduced making calculations of estimated GFR skewed, thus overestimating renal function. Since education is the key element to having more patients on home therapies, a team approach usually works best. The physician rarely has the time to fully educate the patient. Therefore, a patient educator will be instrumental to increasing the use of home dialysis. The educator should have pamphlets, DVDs, and time to visit with the patient and family. Group sessions can also be very helpful. When the patient finds others facing similar life-changing decisions, they realize they are not alone in having to make difficult decisions regarding treatment for renal failure. Using current home patients to provide testimonials can be very helpful. If the patient with progressive renal failure speaks to someone already on a home therapy, they often realize the benefits of home dialysis and the fear of doing a home therapy subsides. The patient often has more confidence in the advice of another patient over marketing brochures. Still marketing material can be helpful and should be available in multiple languages, if possible, so that local ethnic groups can benefit.

Encouraging Home Hemodialysis

For all patients considering dialysis, home hemodialysis should be one of the considerations. As physician, nurses, and health care providers, we have to begin considering home therapies first and in-center treatments second. Home therapies allow patients to live independently. Because funding for dialysis in the future may become more limited, looking to therapies such as home hemodialysis that reduce cost will become more attractive.

Treatments at home can be tailored to the patient. For those patients who struggle with control of their thirst and need frequent dialysis to remove fluid, dialysis in a home setting can be adjusted to manage the fluid gains. Conforming to a 3-day a week schedule does not fit everyone with ESRD. If a patient who normally complies with the diet eats excessive salt or drinks excessive fluid during a special celebration, they can simply dialyze themselves extra to manage this problem. Similarly a diabetic patient who deviates from their diabetic diet and subsequently has high blood sugars adjusts their insulin to accommodate hyperglycemia. We wouldn't want the patient's blood sugars to run high leading to all the consequences of hyperglycemia, but instead we would want the patient to adjust their insulin dosage to lower the blood sugar. In the situation of a renal failure patient with fluid overload, it is prudent to remove the extra fluid and reduce the after load on the heart created by fluid excess. This can be accomplished with home hemodialysis where the extra treatment can be performed by the patient when the need arises.

These types of arguments should be presented to the patient approaching dialysis. Convincing the patient and their family of the value of home hemodialysis takes time and frequent interaction. They have to hear the benefits repeatedly because the idea of starting dialysis can be overwhelming to the patient, particularly if they have never

Table 4.2 Factors of home hemodialysis success

% Success

Factors contributing to Home Hemodialysis Success. (Unpublished raw data)

been told of the options prior to requiring dialysis. The equipment appears threatening to them, the time commitment unmanageable, and the costs insurmountable.

When we looked at our home hemodialysis program, we found that the greatest success was achieved if either the patient or the helper was employed. The next most successful population was the elderly where the patient and the helper are not employed. We had the poorest success if only the patient was solely responsible for the treatment and the partner learned only the basics to handle emergencies. It would appear that the patient needs an advocate who can offer support and help the patient day by day to perform their treatments and give them encouragement (Table 4.2).

Dialysis in Assisted Living Facilities

In the past, it was common for the elderly to be cared for at home through their declining years by their children. Today, however, the elderly often move to assisted living homes when they need help with activities of daily living. Although advantages of home hemodialysis from a clinical standpoint may be obvious, the new home situation may prevent adoption of the home treatment.

Assisted living facilities often charge their guest based on the amount of services needed. For example, if the client needs more assistance with their medications, dressing, or bathing, there may be additional charges. If home hemodialysis of the elderly were permitted in an assisted living environment, the spouse could learn the treatment, but assistance from the nursing staff at the facility could allow and encourage the elderly couple to consider home hemodialysis. While this may lead to an additional charge to the patient by the facility, it could be reasonable if the spouse would perform the majority of the therapy. It could be particularly advantageous to develop assisted living facilities that provide specialized care of the renal failure patient. The home dialysis department could work with the nursing staff of the facility to develop a comprehensive program that would assist with the diet and medications as well as with the treatment itself.

Self-Care

A middle step to home therapy that isn't often used is self-care. Starting a self-care unit where the patient sets up their own machine, sticks their access, and runs on a schedule that allows more flexibility than in-center treatments can be a helpful option. There are currently very few self-care centers in the United States for patients but this option should be expanded to provide more options for the patient. These centers should be staffed with home dialysis nurses who will allow the patient to conduct their own treatments. Often in-center nursing staff have difficulty training elderly patients for home therapies owing to busy schedules and slow learning process. Nursing staff oriented to home therapies will usually have more successful outcomes in such settings.

Summary

The elderly are faced with many difficult problems and decisions as their kidneys fail. Typically the disease that is causing their kidney failure is not confined to the kidneys but often represents a diffuse disease process. This process frequently leads to serious cardiac problems, peripheral vascular disease, and dementia in a body simply failing from age. The elderly often have depression because of their failing health, loss of independence, and the death of loved ones. Independent living facilities and assisted living facilities have filled a gap for those whose families cannot care for their elderly parents. Currently these facilities are often not willing to take on patients performing home dialysis or assist them with their treatments. The

Key Points
1. Elderly patients constitute an ever-growing segment of dialysis population, in the western world.
2. In-center hemodialysis may not be the best option for a significant number of elderly hemodialysis patients.
3. Home therapies are a good alternative for the elderly on dialysis.
4. Home hemodialysis may offer increased flexibility and improved symptom control owing to higher frequency and/or duration of hemodialysis besides being a "gentler" form of therapy.
5. Home hemodialysis machines are becoming increasingly user friendly.
6. Careful patient selection and education remain the key to successful home hemodialysis option for this age group.
7. Transfer from self-care units to home and home hemodialysis in assisted living facilities are under recognized options that are available to elderly patients.

development of specialized assisted living centers that focus on care of the elderly with renal failure may be an attractive option to in-center dialysis.

Home therapies and in particular home hemodialysis have many benefits for the elderly as has been discussed in this chapter. There are, however, many obstacles that must be dealt with to get an elderly patient on home hemodialysis. Using a team of health professionals that includes a social worker, patient educator, home dialysis nurse along with the physician can lead to more patients choosing home hemodialysis.

References

1. U.S. renal data system. USRDS 2005 annual data report: atlas of end-stage renal disease in the United States (2005). National Institutes of Health, National Institute of Diabetes and Digestive and Kidney Diseases, Bethesda
2. List of countries by life expectancy (2010). In: Wikipedia, the free encyclopedia. Retrieved 06 Feb 2013 from http://en.wikipedia.org/w/index.php?title=List_of_countries_by_life_expectancy&oldid=536580534
3. Walls J (1990) Dialysis in the elderly; some U.K. experience. Adv Perit Dial 6:82
4. Dirks JH, Levin NW (2006) Dialysis rationing in South Africa: a global message. Kidney Int 70:982–984
5. Nose Y (1995) Home hemodialysis. A crazy idea in 1963. A memoir. ASAIO J 46:13–17
6. Disney AP (1995) Demography and survival of patients receiving treatment for chronic renal failure in Australia and New Zealand: report on dialysis and renal transplantation treatment from the Australia and New Zealand Dialysis and Transplant Registry. Am J Kidney Dis 25(1):165–175
7. MacGregor MS, Agar JW, Blagg CR (2006) Home haemodialysis – international trends and variation. Nephrol Dial Transplant 21:1934–1945
8. Abdel-Rahman EM, Yan G, Turgut F, Balogun RA (2011) Long-term morbidity and mortality related to falls in hemodialysis patients: role of age and gender – a pilot study. Nephron Clin Pract 118(3):c278–c284
9. Ipema KJ, van der Schans CP, Vok N, deVries JM, Westerhuis R, Duym E, Franssen CF (2012) A difference between day and night: protein intake improves after the transition from conventional to frequent nocturnal hemodialysis. J Ren Nutr 22(3):365–372
10. Hanly PJ, Pierratos A (2001) Improvement of sleep apnea in patients with chronic renal failure who undergo nocturnal hemodialysis. N Engl J Med 344(2):102–107
11. Cornelis T, Kotanko P, Goffin E, Kooman JP, van der Sande FM, Chan CT (2011) Can intensive hemodialysis prevent loss of functionality in the elderly ESRD patient? Semin Dial 24(6):645–652

Chapter 5
Hemodialysis Access in the Elderly: Planning to Execution

Tushar J. Vachharajani

Introduction

The definition of "elderly" is rapidly changing with increasing life span, at least in the developed countries. Being 75 years of age, or above, is commonly accepted definition for an "elderly" and is the fastest growing cohort of end-stage renal disease (ESRD) population. In the United States, since 2000, the adjusted ESRD incident rate among elderly patients has increased by 11 percent [1]. Similarly, a higher incidence of elderly needing dialysis has been seen in other developed countries. The decision to initiate renal replacement therapy in this age group is complex and challenging.

The three most common types of vascular access used in the elderly ESRD patients are arteriovenous fistula (AVF), arteriovenous graft (AVG), and tunneled central venous catheter (CVC). Newer vascular access devices that are available for use in highly selective population are the hemodialysis reliable outflow device (HeRO) and the hybrid vascular graft. The HeRO device is a combination of an expanded polytetrafluoroethylene (ePTFE) graft connected to a silicone-coated outflow component using a titanium connector and is placed across a stenosed central vein. The hybrid vascular graft is made of ePTFE material and uses a sutureless technique to connect the venous end of the conduit thus believed to reduce neointimal hyperplasia and outflow stenosis. The clinical experience with these two newer devices is limited reserving them for patients who have exhausted all other options. A native arteriovenous fistula still remains the most desirable and ideal access in suitable patient.

The suitability of an elderly patient to start hemodialysis and be eligible for AVF creation presumes a significant benefit in both quality and quantity of life. The approach of "fistula first" that is recommended as the "first-choice" dialysis access by several nephrology societies across the globe may not necessarily be the best

T.J. Vachharajani, MD, FASN, FACP
Nephrology Section, W. G. (Bill) Hefner Veterans Affairs Medical Center,
Salisbury, NC, USA
e-mail: tvachh@gmail.com

© Springer Science+Business Media New York 2016   45
M. Misra (ed.), *Dialysis in Older Adults: A Clinical Handbook*,
DOI 10.1007/978-1-4939-3320-4_5

approach in the elderly population. The data on creating a functional AVF in the elderly population is conflicting. The studies have varying definitions for "elderly" and those reporting successful outcomes have the inherent drawback of being retrospective and probably biased in selectively including the healthier elderly patients. Lack of prospective data without selection bias is so far unavailable making it difficult to propose any definitive guidelines. In the elderly patient rather than blindly implementing the "fistula-first" mantra, the process of vascular access planning and its successful execution ought to consider several complex decision-making steps that are outlined below for practical convenience.

Step I   Patient selection for dialysis therapy
Step II   Challenges for effective vascular access planning
Step III   Vascular access selection
Step IV   Vascular access planning
Step V   Effective execution of the plan

Step I: Patient Selection for Dialysis Therapy

Likelihood of Death vs. Progression to Dialysis

The prevalence of chronic kidney disease (CKD) in the elderly population is high, but the progression of the disease is much slower compared to their younger counterparts. The life expectancy in the elderly population can vary significantly, but overall the likelihood of elderly patients needing dialysis therapy is lower compared to death [2]. The high incidence of cardiovascular mortality associated with moderate to severe chronic kidney disease in this age group is well recognized. The very old patients (defined as age more than 85 years) are less likely to need dialysis therapy even with estimated glomerular filtration rates of less than 15 ml/min/1.73 m². Moreover, the very elderly patients who are often frail with poor functional status and multiple comorbidities have 3- to 6-fold greater risk of death [3]. Thus, the CKD management in the elderly necessitates an open discussion about the risks and benefits of initiating hemodialysis therapy. An alternate approach of active medical management (avoiding the term *palliative care*) may be desirable for elderly patients with high comorbidity scores, markedly poor functional status, and relatively short life span. A placement of vascular access in this population may trigger unnecessary procedures leading to poor quality of life increasing pain and morbidity and ultimately contributing to higher healthcare costs [4].

Step II: Challenges for Effective Vascular Access Planning

Arteriovenous fistula remains the preferred access for dialysis even in the elderly population. Guidelines and initiatives from several societies advocate quality benchmarks and suggest practice standards to improve overall quality of care. The intent to achieve these set targets for creating functioning AVF in the incident and prevalent dialysis population are the driving force behind quality measures. Unfortunately, elderly CKD patient fall outside the realm of these "standard of care" guidelines. Vascular access planning brings in unique challenges in the elderly CKD population. The various observational studies reported in literature often fail to address complex issues relevant for vascular access planning in this cohort. Figure 5.1 outlines these relevant patient factors that play an important role in the decision algorithm.

Cardiovascular Disease Burden

Elderly ESRD patients with significant cardiac disease may be vulnerable to cardiac decompensation following a permanent arteriovenous access creation, especially with a high flow upper arm access. The creation of an AVF/AVG with blood flows more than 2 L/min may increase the risk of high-output congestive heart failure. The negative role of higher blood flows on pulmonary hypertension, cardiac output, and ejection fraction has been described. The combination of diabetes mellitus and

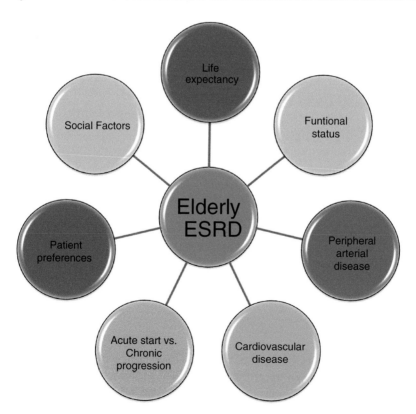

Fig. 5.1 Challenges in an elderly end-stage renal disease (ESRD) patient

poor cardiac function has an additive effect on the overall poor survival in the elderly patients with CKD [5].

The use of cardiac implantable electronic devices (CIED) is on the rise in the elderly CKD patients. The presence of CIED poses several new challenges while planning for a permanent vascular access for dialysis. The presence of such hardware in the central veins increases the potential to develop central vein stenosis especially in combination with a large bore central vein dialysis catheter. The presence of CKD increases the risk for CIED infection and is independent of all other factors. The combination of CKD, CIED, and CVC catheter is worrisome as the risk of catheter-related bacteremia has been reported to be up to 5.5 episodes per 1000 catheter days. The high blood flow from an ipsilateral vascular access as the CIED can potentially unmask the underlying central venous stenosis precipitating clinical symptoms [6].

Functional Status

The cognitive function tends to decline rapidly in the elderly dialysis patient and can shorten the life span significantly [7]. The efforts and resources utilized to create a permanent access in the debilitated elderly population are often unjustified and need careful evaluation.

Peripheral Arterial Disease

Atherosclerotic arterial disease in the elderly patient may hinder the maturation process, and preoperative evaluation can assist with ideal site selection [8]. The presence of significantly small distal arteries may prevent creation of a functional access at the wrist. A complete risk evaluation for developing distal ischemia and steal syndrome post vascular access creation needs to be an integral component of access planning. Arterial and venous calcification has been described in about a third of the vessels used for creating vascular access. The amount of calcification is known to worsen with progressing CKD and age, resulting in poor maturation of arteriovenous fistula.

Patient Preference

An elderly patient with CKD nearing dialysis is often faced with multiple social and moral issues, which may play a role in their final selection of vascular access. A strong sense of guilt, an attitude of extending life "one day at a time," and sense of burden imposed on their caregivers may drive the elderly to choose CVC over a permanent vascular access. Additionally, fear of needles and associated pain may tilt the balance in favor of CVC over AVF/AVG. Patients who are already on dialysis may form their own opinion based on patient-patient interactions, personal experience, and observations in the dialysis unit [9].

Acute Start vs. Chronic Progression

The development of an acute need to initiate hemodialysis is not uncommon in clinical practice. Timely access planning may not be an option in relatively stable elderly CKD patients with high comorbidities, who often deteriorate rapidly while being admitted for non-renal diseases. The use of CVC in patients requiring acute start is unavoidable, but the goal should be to transition them to a permanent access as soon as the clinical condition improves.

Socioeconomic Factors

Elderly patients depend on others for their healthcare visits. Typically, creating a permanent vascular access involves visits for vessel mapping, preoperative anesthesia clearance, surgery, and follow-up evaluations. These visits can lead to loss of productivity for the caregiver contributing to the ultimate decision.

Step III: Vascular Access Selection

AVF vs. AVG

Arteriovenous fistula remains the preferred vascular access in the younger CKD population because of the lower incidence of infection, stenosis, and thrombosis resulting in overall longer patency compared to AVG and CVC. The clinical experience and outcomes of AVF are not necessarily identical in the elderly CKD patient [10]. There is a higher incidence of fistula maturation failure due to small, calcified, and atherosclerotic vessels. The patency rates for AVF reported in literature vary widely because of the variability in definitions and selection bias and practice patterns. Figure 5.2 outlines the critical factors that play a significant role in the AVF maturation process.

Arteriovenous grafts are considered the second best option, especially with multiple failed AVFs, with unsuitable or damaged veins, and to limit the duration of CVC use. AVGs have a lower patency rate and higher associated morbidity related to frequent development of stenosis and thrombotic events. The patency data available in the literature on AVG in the elderly patient is not robust and with high variability making it difficult to draw definitive conclusions.

The interpretation of patency data reported in literature comparing AVF and AVG is dependent on the definitions used in the study. The overall cumulative patency of AVF and AVG is identical when the primary non-maturing AVF is included in the survival analysis [11]. A survival analysis from the US Renal Data System on the type of vascular access in >65–year-old did not reveal any advantage between AVF and AVG. The cumulative patency was identical in elderly patients with and without diabetes, and in fact, AVG survival was better compared to AVF in the first 18 months after access creation.

Site Selection: Forearm vs. Upper Arm

The consensus guidelines from several societies recommend radiocephalic AVF as the first-choice vascular access. The fistula maturation failure in the elderly population, especially of the radiocephalic fistula, is higher compared to the younger counterparts. In a meta-analysis of 13 studies, the patency rate for radiocephalic and brachiocephalic fistula was reduced equally in the elderly patients. In a secondary analysis, the 12-month patency rate of brachiocephalic AVF was higher by 12 %

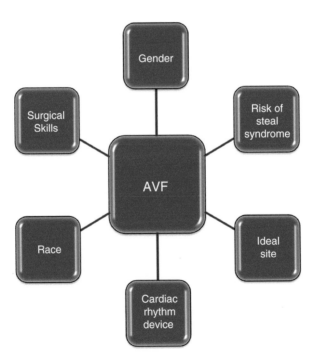

Fig. 5.2 Factors influencing maturation of an arteriovenous fistula (AVF)

compared to radiocephalic AVF [12]. The available data for 1-year and 5-year cumulative survival of AVF in the elderly remains conflicting compared to younger ESRD patients.

Central Venous Catheter

Limiting the use of CVC remains the best option given its associated higher morbidity and mortality compared to AVF/AVG. CVC can be considered as an acceptable primary access in the elderly CKD patients with: (i) short life expectancy, (ii) acute start dialysis, (iii) chronic hypotension making it difficult to support prescribed blood flows for adequate dialysis therapy, (iv) severe peripheral vascular disease posing a surgical challenge for access creation, and (v) complications like steal syndrome and risk of distal ischemia and (vi) during a limited time trial before deciding on long-term commitment and (vii) all possible vascular access sites have been exhausted.

Step IV: Vascular Access Planning

Vascular access planning is time consuming and needs active participation of several members. Figure 5.3 outlines the various team members and patient factors that need to be considered while selecting an ideal vascular access for an elderly patient

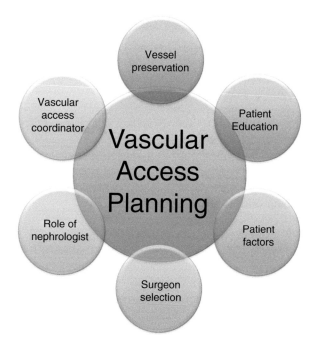

Fig. 5.3 Key factors in the vascular access planning process

with CKD. Besides the patient, the vascular access planning team should include a vascular access coordinator/educator, a nephrologist, and a competent surgeon. Patient education plays a very important role in the entire planning process. The role of the educator/coordinator is to educate the patient and family members the importance of taking a timely decision and the pros and cons of different vascular access options. The education process should also involve explaining the goals and expectations from dialysis therapy and the necessary change it can bring to the lifestyle of both the patient and their family members. The nephrologist and the surgeon should take in to consideration all the challenges and patient-related factors discussed above to decide on creating an ideal vascular access for each individual patient. The vascular access coordinator then assists in facilitating and implementing the plan so the desired vascular access is created long before the actual need for dialysis therapy.

Step V: Effective Execution of the Plan

Evaluate Comorbidities

A thorough evaluation and documentation of comorbidities is essential once the decision is made to prepare a patient for hemodialysis therapy. A detailed history pertaining to previous CVC and failed attempts at permanent accesses should be documented. Patients with CIED should be identified for objective evaluation of the central vein patency before being referred to a surgeon.

Evaluation of Vessels

Vascular access is a circuit that Starts and ends at the heart and includes the peripheral arterial and the venous system of the extremity. Evaluating the arteries and veins for ideal site selection is important to minimize maturation failure. The vessels can be evaluated with physical examination, Doppler ultrasonography, venogram, and if necessary selective arteriogram studies.

Physical examination is a simple bedside tool that can provide valuable information for suitability of both artery and vein in creating an AVF. A modified Allen test performed using pulse oximetry signal can assist in identifying elderly patients at risk of developing steal syndrome.

Doppler ultrasonography can simultaneously help evaluate the arteries and superficial veins. The compliance and distensibility of superficial veins can be assessed with and without the use of a tourniquet. Doppler ultrasonography has a distinct advantage over venography as it also allows evaluation of the arteries for the presence of calcification and blood flow assessment, without the potential risk of precipitating contrast-related nephropathy. Venography has its role in evaluating the central veins in high-risk patients especially those with multiple previous CVC or with a CIED.

A minimum venous luminal diameter of 2.5 mm and arterial diameter of 2.0 mm are considered favorable for suitable vascular access creation. Even though these criteria are commonly used in clinical practice, successful fistula maturation process remains unpredictable. In older women, primary AVF failure rate has been reported to be as high as 78 % despite vessel mapping [13].

Surgical Skills

The surgical training and skills have been shown to be important to create a successful vascular access. The selection of a dedicated, skilled, and innovative surgeon in the vascular access team can improve the success of the vascular access program.

Interventionalist

An interventionalist can be a nephrologist, radiologist, or a vascular surgeon and remains an integral member of the vascular access team [14]. An interventionalist plays a vital role in the evaluation of non-maturing AVFs and treats failing accesses with endovascular procedures. Endovascular procedures remain the mainstay therapy to maintain the access patency. The procedures are commonly performed in an outpatient setting and prevent loss of dialysis treatment. There is a growing trend across the globe for nephrologists to take a leadership role in patient selection, planning, and performing endovascular procedures and act as a liaison between the dialysis units and the surgeons.

Summary: Individualized Approach

Vascular access creation in an elderly CKD patient is clearly a challenging process and involves a complex multistep process. The vascular access planning should start with an open discussion about risks and benefits of initiating dialysis therapy giving equal consideration for quality of life rather than quantity of life. The discussion should include not only the patient but also the family members and consider alternate treatment modalities such as peritoneal dialysis or active non-dialysis medical therapy. A common sense approach is sometimes the "best approach," and incorporating life expectancy, functional status, relevant comorbidities, and available surgical expertise can guide the ideal vascular access creation process. Even though guidelines suggest "fistula-first" approach, in the elderly CKD population "patient-first" approach may be more rational. A suggested algorithm for an individualized approach as provided in Fig. 5.4 may be a practical way until more definitive data are available to guide practice patterns [15].

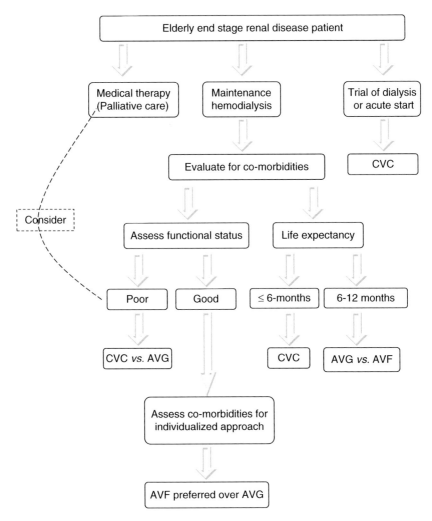

Fig. 5.4 Suggested algorithm for an individualized approach to dialysis vascular access planning in an elderly patient with chronic kidney disease

Key Points
1. Vascular access planning in elderly ESRD requires multidisciplinary team involvement and poses unique challenges.
2. Multiple comorbidities, complex social circumstances, patient preferences, and quality of life issues dictate the decision-making process.
3. Arteriovenous fistula remains the preferred long-term vascular access but may not be an ideal vascular access for all elderly ESRD patients.
    Active medical management (palliative care), peritoneal dialysis, and end-of-life care therapies should be offered to elderly ESRD as treatment options.

References

1. U.S. Renal Data System (2009) USRDS 2009 Annual Report: atlas of end-stage renal disease in the United States, National Institutes of Health, National Institute of Diabetes and Digestive and Kidney Diseases, Bethesda
2. Joly D, Anglicheau D, Alberti C et al (2003) Octogenarians reaching end-stage renal disease: cohort study of decision-making and clinical outcomes. J Am Soc Nephrol JASN 14(4):1012–1021
3. O'Hare AM, Choi AI, Bertenthal D et al (2007) Age affects outcomes in chronic kidney disease. J Am Soc Nephrol JASN 18(10):2758–2765
4. Moist LM, Lok CE, Vachharajani TJ et al (2012) Optimal hemodialysis vascular access in the elderly patient. Semin Dial 25(6):640–648
5. Basile C, Lomonte C, Vernaglione L, Casucci F, Antonelli M, Losurdo N (2008) The relationship between the flow of arteriovenous fistula and cardiac output in haemodialysis patients. Nephrol Dial Transplant Off Publ Eur Dial Transplant Assoc Eur Renal Assoc 23(1):282–287
6. Asif A, Salman L, Lopera G, Haqqie SS, Carrillo R (2012) Transvenous cardiac implantable electronic devices and hemodialysis catheters: recommendations to curtail a potentially lethal combination. Semin Dial 25(5):582–586
7. Kurella M, Covinsky KE, Collins AJ, Chertow GM (2007) Octogenarians and nonagenarians starting dialysis in the United States. Annals of Internal Medicine 146(3):177–183
8. Lok CE, Oliver MJ, Su J, Bhola C, Hannigan N, Jassal SV (2005) Arteriovenous fistula outcomes in the era of the elderly dialysis population. Kidney International 67(6):2462–2469
9. Xi W, Harwood L, Diamant MJ et al (2011) Patient attitudes towards the arteriovenous fistula: a qualitative study on vascular access decision making. Nephrol Dial Transplant Off Publ Eur Dial Transplant Assoc Eur Renal Assoc 26(10):3302–3308
10. Feldman HI, Joffe M, Rosas SE, Burns JE, Knauss J, Brayman K (2003) Predictors of successful arteriovenous fistula maturation. Am J Kidney Dis Off J Natl Kidney Found 42(5):1000–1012
11. Allon M, Lok CE (2010) Dialysis fistula or graft: the role for randomized clinical trials. Clin J Am Soc Nephrol CJASN 5(12):2348–2354
12. Lazarides MK, Georgiadis GS, Antoniou GA, Staramos DN (2007) A meta-analysis of dialysis access outcome in elderly patients. J Vascu Surg 45(2):420–426
13. Peterson WJ, Barker J, Allon M (2008) Disparities in fistula maturation persist despite preoperative vascular mapping. Clin J Am Soc Nephrol CJASN 3(2):437–441
14. Vachharajani TJ, Moossavi S, Salman L et al (2011) Dialysis vascular access management by interventional nephrology programs at University Medical Centers in the United States. Seminars in Dialysis 24(5):564–569
15. Vachharajani T (2011) Dialysis vascular access selection in elderly patients. Eur Nephrol 5(2):152–154

Chapter 6
Peritoneal Dialysis for the Elderly

Edwina A. Brown

Introduction

The default dialysis choice for the elderly is usually haemodialysis in most European countries, Canada and the USA with relatively few patients starting on peritoneal dialysis (PD) compared to younger and fitter patients. This is actually quite surprising as a home-based treatment avoids the need for transport and peritoneal dialysis (PD) does not have the haemodynamic swings associated with haemodialysis (HD). There is no doubt that there are often challenges to enabling an elderly patient to have PD, but the development of assisted PD can surmount many of these. Indeed, in France where assisted PD has been available for many years, the PD population is predominantly elderly [1]. As discussed in Chap. 2, the BOLDE study has shown that PD patients have less illness and treatment intrusion than patients on HD [2], though the patients in the BOLDE study were mainly fitter older patients and none were on assisted PD.

Eligibility for PD

PD eligibility for older patients depends on factors related to the PD itself and on those more specifically related to ageing (see Table 16.1). Older patients are also more likely to be late presenters or "crashlanders". Once started on HD, they are often unlikely to change to PD. With planning and appropriate education, many of the barriers can be surmounted. With appropriate education, over half of older patients would prefer to be on PD [3]. In this study of 134 older incident Canadian

E.A. Brown
Imperial Renal and Transplant Centre, Hammersmith Hospital,
Du Cane Road, London W12 0HS, UK
e-mail: e.a.brown@imperial.ac.uk

© Springer Science+Business Media New York 2016
M. Misra (ed.), *Dialysis in Older Adults: A Clinical Handbook*,
DOI 10.1007/978-1-4939-3320-4_6

Table 6.1 Potential obstacles for PD in elderly patients

	Potential obstacle	Solution
PD related	Prior lower abdominal surgery	Consider surgically placed catheter, but PD may be contraindicated, particularly in presence of colostomy, previous pelvic radiotherapy, etc.
	Severe obesity	Consider surgically placed catheter but PD may be contraindicated
	Housing – no storage space	Can be a contraindication, but consider more frequent smaller deliveries of supplies
	Depression/anxiety	Can be a contraindication, but consider assisted PD
Age-related	Poor manual dexterity	Consider assisted PD
	Impaired physical activity with difficulty in lifting bags of fluid	Consider assisted PD
	Impaired vision	Consider assisted PD
	Impaired hearing	Use visual aids for training; consider assisted PD
	Cognitive dysfunction	Consider assisted PD. Can be contraindication if patient gets agitated, at risk of contaminating catheter or exit site
	General frailty	Consider assisted PD
	Late presentation (more common in elderly)	Consider acute start PD ± assisted PD

patients with a median age of 73 years, 25 % had visual problems, 20 % were considered immobile and 17 % had reduced hearing. In units with assisted PD available, 80 % patients were deemed eligible for PD as against 65 % when assistance was not available. In both groups, almost 60 % of those eligible chose PD. Oliver et al. [4] have also shown how important social support is for the eventual choice of PD; family support was associated with an increase in PD eligibility from 63 to 80 % and PD choice from 40 to 57 % in patients with barriers to self-care.

Benefits of PD for Older Patients

The advantages and disadvantages of PD compared to HD for older patients are discussed in Chap. 2. As shown in Table 16.2, the principal advantage of PD is being able to have treatment at home and thereby avoid the disruption and discomfort of visits to hospital in all weathers and regardless of how the patient is feeling. Furthermore, PD avoids the haemodynamic swings associated with HD and enables more freedom in terms of travel. This can be particularly important for older people who wish to visit family members in different parts of the world. Finally, and a point that is often not considered, there is the benefit of preservation of residual renal function enabling a relatively low dialysis prescription which minimises treatment burden and intrusion into lifestyle. It is well recognised that rate of decline in kidney function is lower with increasing age. Calculation of PD clearance includes residual

Table 6.2 Benefits of PD for older patients

Treatment is at home
Hospital visits restricted to outpatient reviews and emergency visits
Flexibility of treatment times round social activities (CAPD) or at night with daytime freedom (APD)
Preservation of residual renal function enabling 1–2 days "off"/week and slow incremental dose of treatment
No haemodynamic swings so stable blood pressure and no periods of feeling "washed out" (as compared to HD)
Simple procedure so can be done by family member or paid assistant with minimal training time

renal function, thereby enabling an incremental increase in the PD prescription as renal function declines; if there is little decline, dose of PD remains low. It is therefore not uncommon to find older patients still using only 3 CAPD exchanges some years after starting dialysis.

Assisted PD

Realistically, very few frail elderly patients will be able to perform their own PD. In some instances, family members will help, but usually, when this is not possible, patients are placed on HD with all its difficulties, and a few will opt for conservative care, i.e., no dialysis. Patients incapable of self-care PD, however, could be supported through assisted peritoneal dialysis (aPD) where trained staff provides daily dialysis assistance either in nursing homes or in patients' homes. Assisted PD is available in many European countries, in parts of Canada and Australia using healthcare workers and in many Asian and South American countries where domestic help is often relatively inexpensive. Assisted PD, however, is not reimbursed in the USA and so is not readily available unless provided by the patient and/or their family.

French Experience: Assisted CAPD

In France, aPD has been standard treatment for older patients for many years. A detailed analysis by the French REIN registry [5] of 3512 patients over 75 years starting dialysis between 2002 and 2005 showed that 18 % began with PD, with the proportion varying from 3 to 38 % depending on region; over half of these patients were on assisted PD. Interestingly, starting dialysis with PD was significantly associated with older age, congestive heart failure and severe behavioural disorders. The availability of assistance has enabled PD in France to be predominantly a treatment of the elderly, with ~55 % of patients on PD in January 2011 being >70 years of age

[1]. Non-disconnect CAPD with UV flash is the predominant method used as this greatly shortens the time needed for the nurse visit—the nurse phones the patient or a relative to start the drain procedure so when he/she arrives, they just have to remove the old bag and connect the new one, leaving the fluid to drain in and the patient to fold up the bag after their departure.

Assisted APD

In other European countries and in Canada, APD is used as the PD modality for assisted patients. Table 16.3 shows different models of how this is delivered.

Training of Assistants

Length of time taken to train assistants depends on healthcare experience of that individual. If a family member or a layperson provided by the patient or family, then training is no different to the standard training provided by the PD team for patients starting treatment. Nurses usually only require about half a day's training in the PD unit. In the UK system, assistants are mostly provided through a healthcare agency and require a longer period of training which is done either by the local PD unit or in a commercial PD training unit. In all programmes, the local PD team need to provide backup and be available for advice for the PD assistant.

Table 6.3 Models of delivering assisted APD

Europe (non-UK), Canada
Community nurses visit twice a day
Morning visit to disconnect patient from cycler machine, remove used bags and set up machine with new bags for the evening
Shorter evening visit to connect patient to cycler machine
This model is being developed in some European countries (Sweden, Denmark, Netherlands, Belgium, France) and Canada
Main disadvantage is cost of using nurses and providing 2 visits/day
UK
Daily visit from a healthcare assistant (individual with short basic training in healthcare)
Nursing qualification is not needed to perform PD (usually done by patients ± family support); salary of healthcare assistant is less than a nurse
One visit a day only – assistant takes used bags off cycler machine and sets up machine with new bags and also checks blood pressure and weight of patient and can perform exit site dressings
Patient (with or without family support) still has to do their own connection to and disconnection from the cycler machine. This limits the patient population suitable for assisted PD

Selection of Patients for Assisted PD

Patients starting on assisted PD come from various sources: existing PD patients who are no longer able to perform autonomous PD, predialysis patients starting dialysis electively, patients who have chosen PD but are difficult to train and HD patients who tolerate HD poorly. Assisted PD is also useful for patients who present late and are started on PD acutely ("acute-start PD") while they wait for a training slot or to provide a transition period during which they can adjust to life on dialysis.

Not all elderly patients are suitable for aPD. Apart from the standard contraindications to PD, factors that make patients unsuitable for aPD include restlessness at night so unable to stay on machine, living alone and unable to be trained for eventuality of machine alarming overnight (if necessary, response can be just to switch off machine), unable to be trained to disconnect from machine in emergency, accommodation too small for cycling machine and fluid supplies and patient proves to be unreliable so frequently not at home when assistant calls.

Quality of Life

Anecdotally, patients can be very stable on aPD and those who have transferred from HD feel much better. There are currently no studies which report specifically on quality of life in patients on assisted PD.

Management of PD

Management of patients on PD includes initial assessment, catheter insertion, training and maintenance. The majority of the principles of care are the same as for younger patients, but there are features that need to be highlighted for older patients.

Assessment for PD

Apart from standard assessment for PD eligibility, older patients need to be assessed for their physical ability to carry out the various procedures required and for the ability to learn how to perform these techniques and how to troubleshoot if things go wrong. As already discussed, they are more likely to have poor hand dexterity, difficulty in lifting heavy bags, cognitive dysfunction (particularly impaired executive function), impaired vision and impaired hearing. All these factors will create difficulties in performing PD independently. Particularly when problems are anticipated, the PD assessment should be carried out in the patient's home and with their family or carer support present. Potential barriers can then be identified and appropriate social support can be suggested to the family and/or put in place with community support. Some patients may benefit from creation of a microenvironment, enabling them to carry out PD independently. As well as identifying physical problems, it is also important to identify whether patients can carry over information and to obtain information from family or carers about potential memory or other cognitive problems. If it appears unlikely that the patient will be able to carry out their own PD, the possibility of assisted PD either by the family or a paid healthcare worker should be discussed at this stage.

Catheter Insertion

There is no evidence of increased complications from catheter insertion such as hernia or fluid leak in older patients. In terms of actual insertion, as older patients are more likely to have cardiovascular comorbidities, it is important to assess suitability for general anaesthetic if this is going to be needed for catheter insertion.

Patient Training

If the patient has been assessed appropriately prior to PD catheter insertion, potential difficulties such as poor hand dexterity and impaired vision or hearing should have been identified. As many older patients do have impaired hearing and find learning more difficult, training should be done in a quiet environment and can take longer than for younger patients. Aids to learning, such as pictures, are often helpful. The most common problem in training older patients is previously undiagnosed cognitive impairment. This is much more common in patients with chronic kidney disease than in the general population, and executive function is often more severely affected than memory. It is hardly surprising, therefore, that such patients find it difficult to learn how to do their own PD. For a patient who appears difficult or impossible to train, the options are finding a family member to help, providing assistance at home or changing to haemodialysis.

Maintenance on PD

Maintaining any patient on PD is a multi-professional activity. For the elderly, holistic care is vitally important. As well as all the features of usual dialysis care, one needs to consider the management and progression of the associated comorbidities and impact of general ageing. A patient may be able to cope independently when starting on PD but, with the development of cognitive impairment and/or worsening physical function, may need considerable support and/or be unable to carry out their own PD later on. Decisions then need to be made about social support at home, whether PD continues to be possible or not and whether changing to HD would be beneficial or not. Provision of assisted PD can often enable patients to remain on PD. Regular conversations are essential with patients and families to update on prognosis and determine wishes regarding future care, both regarding need for social support and assistance for PD and end of life planning. When discussing possible transfer to HD, it is important to be realistic about life on HD that such a transfer will not improve comorbidities or the effects of ageing. It is also important to be aware of the impact of PD on families, particularly if the patient is dependent on their spouse, who is most likely also going to be elderly with their own health problems. Temporary periods of assistance may well be needed during periods of illness of the spouse or to give the family a break; this may entail training another family member to do PD, providing paid assistance, or temporary intermittent PD in the hospital.

Complications of PD

There is no evidence of PD-related complications being more common in older patients. Although there has been concern that peritonitis is more frequent in the elderly, this has not been confirmed in most studies. Even with assisted PD in the frail elderly, the French experience shows very acceptable peritonitis rates of 1/36 patient months with nurse assistance and 1/48 patient months with family assistance [6]. There is no evidence of increased risk of hernias or leaks in older patients. There has been no comparison of rate of decline of residual renal function in older compared to younger patients on PD and therefore the risk of problems related to anuria. It is well recognised, though, that rate of decline of renal function is slower with increasing age. It is therefore not uncommon to find older patients continuing to pass urine and have significant residual renal function for up to many years on PD.

Length of Time on PD

Concerns about limiting length of time on PD for older patients should not be an issue. Even after 5 years on PD, the risk of encapsulating peritoneal sclerosis (EPS) is only 5 %. Given the short survival of older patients on dialysis (median survival for patients >75 years old is only 22 months in the UK), if they survive for 5 years on dialysis, they have done well. Transferring to HD at some arbitrary time period would have a major impact on lifestyle and quality of life, could well be deleterious in terms of progression of cognitive dysfunction and physical function and actually increases the risk of developing EPS.

End of Life Management

Dialysis, of any sort, should be regarded as palliative treatment for older patients and particularly for the frail. Life expectancy is considerably shortened and death should not come as a surprise. A realistic prognosis should therefore be discussed with patients and families so that they can express their wishes and achieve end of life goals. Many patients choosing a home therapy would prefer to die at home. This will often require joint management with the palliative care team with care focused on symptom control rather than achieving ideal blood result targets. Withdrawal of dialysis is often less of an issue than for patients on HD as families/carers can be advised that missing an exchange or a night on cycler is acceptable if the patient is drowsy or not well. This is less traumatic than deciding that dialysis is going to stop on a specific day. Care of PD patients requires community support and holistic care. The PD multidisciplinary team is therefore well placed to provide end of life support, interact with community care and palliative care and thereby maximise the quality of life at the end of life for their patients. At the end of life, supporting the patient with social care and symptom control is more important than achieving dialysis targets.

The complexity of caring for an elderly patient on PD is illustrated by the following case history.

Case History

Edith started PD at age 71 years. She had presented with vomiting and found to have end-stage kidney disease with an eGFR of 8 ml/min/1.73 m^2. Her only past history was a cerebellar stroke 10 years previously which had left her with impaired balance so that she walked with a roller zimmer frame. She greatly valued her independence, lived on her own and did all her own activities of daily living. She had never married and her only relative was a brother who lived some distance away; they phoned each other a couple of times a year but had not met for some time. She was maintained on CAPD 3 exchanges/day and did very well for the first 2 years. She continued to be independent, was always smart when coming to the clinic and had no episodes of peritonitis. She then started having falls when outside and in the house. Her walking improved after some physiotherapy and fortunately she had no fractures. After 3 years on PD, it was obvious that she was not coping so well. However she refused to have any help at home and soldiered on. Conversations were had about the future – she was always adamant that she did not want to change to HD and that she did not want a lingering death; she had seen her sister die from a brain tumour over many months and did not want the same for herself. The inevitable crisis happened when she came to the clinic fluid overloaded, anaemic and clearly not dialysing. She admitted to falling asleep and missing exchanges. She now agreed to change to assisted APD. At the community visit to set this up, it was obvious that she no longer cleaned her house and had not been eating. It proved impossible to train her how to turn alarms off on the cycler machine and it became apparent that she was now significantly cognitively impaired. After 1 week of assisted APD, she was reviewed in the clinic. She appeared dishevelled with food stains on her clothes; she had bruises on her face and abdomen but could not remember falling. Although her memory was clearly poor, she was still clear that she did not want HD, but she did not want to stop dialysis. As she retained the ability to do CAPD exchanges, the plan was changed to increasing social support at home with carers visiting regularly, meals on wheels were organised and she returned to do CAPD with the realisation that she would often miss an exchange. Community palliative care was also organised to provide nurse support at home and to enable her to transfer to a hospice when clinically indicated.

Key Points

1. Peritoneal dialysis should be considered for all older patients considering dialysis to enable treatment at home.
2. Assisted peritoneal dialysis is provided by many healthcare systems and enables older patients to have dialysis at home even when they cannot undertake treatment themselves.
3. No evidence of increased risk of PD-related complications, such as infection, for older patients.
4. Important to provide appropriate psychosocial support for ageing-related factors such as physical and cognitive function decline.
5. Important to discuss overall prognosis and end of life planning with patients and families.

References

1. http://www.rdplf.org/profils/542-profil-2012.html. Accessed 14th Jan 2013
2. Brown EA, Johansson L, Farrington K, Gallagher H, Sensky T, Gordon F, da Silva-Gane M, Beckett N, Hickson M (2010) Broadening Options for Long-term Dialysis for the Elderly (BOLDE): differences in quality of life on peritoneal dialysis compared to haemodialysis for older patients. Nephrol Dial Transplant 25:3755–3763
3. Oliver MJ, Quinn RR, Richardson EP, Kiss AJ, Lamping DL, Manns BJ (2007) Home care assistance and the utilization of peritoneal dialysis. Kidney Int 71:673–678
4. Oliver MJ, Garg AX, Blake PG, Johnson JF, Verrelli M, Zacharias JM, Pandeya S, Quinn RR (2010) Impact of contraindications, barriers to self-care and support on incident peritoneal dialysis utilization. Nephrol Dial Transplant 25:2737–2744
5. Couchoud C, Moranne O, Frimat L, Labeeuw M, Allot V, Stengel B (2007) Associations between comorbidities, treatment choice and outcome in the elderly with end-stage renal disease. Nephrol Dial Transplant 22:3246–3254
6. Verger C, Duman M, Durand PY, Veniez G, Fabre E, Ryckelynck JP (2007) Influence of autonomy and type of home assistance on the prevention of peritonitis in assisted automated peritoneal dialysis patients. An analysis of data from the French Language Peritoneal Dialysis Registry. Nephrol Dial Transplant 22:1218–1222

Chapter 7
Managing Blood Pressure in the Elderly: What Is Different?

Sergio F.F. Santos, George Sunny Pazhayattil, and Aldo J. Peixoto

Introduction

Blood pressure (BP) management is essential in patients with end-stage kidney disease (ESKD) on maintenance dialysis as hypertension is the most common cardiovascular risk factor in this population. Even though this is true across all age groups, the aging process adds challenges to the evaluation and management of BP in dialysis patients. In this chapter, we will review aspects related to the management of BP and the treatment of hypertension in patients on chronic maintenance dialysis, with a focus on issues that are modified by the aging process, being mindful of the caveat that data restricted to elderly patients are scanty.

Epidemiology

The relationship between BP and outcomes in dialysis patients is complex. Many observational studies have shown an inverse relationship between BP and mortality in HD patients [1]. Fewer studies are available in PD cohorts, but the available literature shows similar results [2]. In summary, these studies suggest that the lowest mortality rates in HD patients occur with BP in the range that would be classified as hypertension in the general population (140–160/70–90 mmHg). In these observational studies, the highest mortality rates occur in patients with BP below 120/80 mmHg. Increased mortality in the high BP ranges is only observed when BP is above 180/100 mmHg. With relevance to the elderly, a recent cohort study noted

S.F.F. Santos, MD, PhD
Division of Nephrology, State University of Rio de Janeiro, Rio de Janeiro, Brazil

G.S. Pazhayattil, MD • A.J. Peixoto, MD (✉)
Section of Nephrology, Yale University School of Medicine, New Haven, CT, USA
e-mail: aldo.peixoto@yale.edu

© Springer Science+Business Media New York 2016
M. Misra (ed.), *Dialysis in Older Adults: A Clinical Handbook*,
DOI 10.1007/978-1-4939-3320-4_7

this pattern to be more pronounced in the elderly [3]; in other words, *the older the patient group, the greater the impact of low BP on mortality risk, especially among those aged 70 and older.* In patients under age 60, low BP was not associated with increased risk. These findings raise concern that aggressive BP control in dialysis patients, particularly the elderly, could put them at risk for worse outcomes and certainly complicate efforts to establish BP targets (see below).

There are several possible explanations for this apparent paradox [1, 4]. The most commonly raised is that low BP is associated with congestive heart failure and other severe comorbidities and these observational studies are uniformly flawed by the absence of adjustment for cardiac function. In the only observational study where echocardiographic data were available, no such U-shaped relationship was noted [5]. In addition, there may be a time lag bias; patients have a high mortality in the early stages after initiation of dialysis due to other reasons, and patients with higher BP may take several years to have an impact of high BP levels on mortality. Lastly, there may be a role of the type of BP measurement used, as studies using 48-h ambulatory or home BP monitoring have identified a direct relationship between BP and mortality, differently from BP values obtained in the dialysis unit.

Approximately 90 % of patients with chronic kidney disease have a diagnosis of hypertension by the time they reach ESKD. Contemporary cross-sectional surveys indicate the prevalence of uncontrolled hypertension in hemodialysis (HD) patients to be ~70 %. Similar estimates apply to patients undergoing peritoneal dialysis (PD) (60–90 %) [2, 4]. Interestingly and contrary to what is observed in the general population, the prevalence of hypertension in dialysis patients has no linear relationship with age. Some reports reflect on the very low prevalence of hypertension among patients receiving daily HD, long nocturnal HD, and in selected populations undergoing conventional HD or PD while adhering to aggressive salt restriction. We are not aware of data exploring an interaction between age and blood pressure (BP) in these very selected populations.

Unfortunately, limited clinical trial data are available to isolate the effects of BP lowering as beneficial or detrimental in dialysis patients, and all clinical trials have been underpowered to answer this question. However, two meta-analyses have compiled results from clinical trials in HD patients [6, 7]. In these trials, active antihypertensive drug treatment resulted in BP that was 4.5/2.7 mmHg lower than in the control group. Aggregate results that include both hypertensive and normotensive patients indicate a decrease in risk of death or cardiovascular events of ~20–29 % among patients receiving active treatment. As one would expect, this effect was more prominent among patients who have hypertension (51 % risk reduction). Results from these meta-analyses, while not conclusive, dispel some of the concerns clinicians may have about treating hypertension in dialysis patients. We do not have specific trial data restricted to elderly patients.

Pathophysiology of Hypertension

The pathophysiology of hypertension in dialysis patients is complex, and there are a variety of factors contributing to it. Table 7.1 outlines some of the known factors involved.

Table 7.1 Factors contributing to pathogenesis of hypertension in dialysis patients

Sodium and water retention leading to extracellular volume expansion
Excessive vasoconstriction:
↑Renin-angiotensin system activity
↑Sympathetic nervous system activity
↑Ouabain-like factor
↑Vasopressin
↑Endothelin-1
Decreased vasodilation:
↓Nitric oxide
↓Kinins
Increased intracellular calcium
Increased arterial stiffness
Obstructive sleep apnea
Hyperparathyroidism
Erythropoietin therapy
Renovascular disease

Extracellular Volume Overload

This is the most common and most recognized reason for hypertension in dialysis patients. Increased extracellular fluid (ECF) volume measured with different methods is associated with increased BP levels, and that seems to be *more pronounced in older patients* [8]. Patients receiving daily or prolonged HD reach better BP control at least in part through improved ECF volume status, though other mechanisms are likely operative as well. In a randomized clinical trial in patients receiving conventional HD, increased ultrafiltration resulting in a 1 kg difference in dry weight between groups translated into a 6.6/3.3 mmHg reduction in BP over a 2-month period [9]. In PD patients, patients with peritoneal membrane characteristics leading to faster solute transport are predisposed to volume overload and hypertension [2]. In such patients, improvement of sodium balance with better ultrafiltration (e.g., through the use of icodextrin) results in lower BP levels. Likewise, sodium restriction is associated with improved BP levels in hypertensive HD and PD patients. Overall, volume excess is an important mediator of hypertension in dialysis patients and is particularly relevant because of it can be manipulated clinically in order to lower BP.

Imbalance Between Vasoconstrictive and Vasodilatory Systems

This is a complex area of research involving multiple pathways, and to date, all the elements at play are incompletely understood, but it is apparent that as noted in Table 7.1, several vasoconstrictor systems are commonly overactive in ESKD, whereas vasodilating mechanisms are typically blunted [4, 10]. Of relevance to therapy, the renin-angiotensin system is not usually overactive but fails to suppress in the face of the attendant volume overload. In addition, intrarenal renin activity is markedly increased in dialysis patients. Also of relevance is the well-demonstrated overactivity of the sympathetic nervous system, including output from renal afferents. This can be manipulated pharmacologically and, more recently, with renal sympathetic denervation.

Role of Dialysate Prescription in HD

Dialysate concentration of sodium, calcium, magnesium, and potassium all have effects on intradialytic BP in HD patients [10]. BP increases upon exposure to high sodium or calcium and falls when the dialysate is high in potassium or magnesium. The impact of interdialytic BP is less clearly defined, though it appears that high sodium and calcium also have an effect on longer-term BP control. These observations have impact on treatment decisions (see below). The impact of dialysate composition on BP in PD patients has been less adequately studied, although the role of sodium and calcium appears similar to what is observed in HD.

Arterial Stiffness

Arterial stiffness is accelerated by kidney disease, and patients on dialysis have among the highest degrees of arterial stiffness [11]. This process is mediated largely by increased arterial wall calcification and decreased elastin content. Although aging is associated with arterial stiffening, the strength of this relationship is blunted in patients on dialysis. Arterial stiffness results in increased pulse wave velocity, which causes an increase in central arterial pressure as a consequence of faster reflection of pulse waves. BP lowering through any means but particularly through control of sodium excess and use of blockers of the renin-angiotensin system is an effective way of decreasing pulse wave velocity. However, there are no proven strategies to improve the fundamental abnormalities of the arterial wall.

The other mechanistic factors listed in Table 7.1 are also operative in some cases and need to be entertained as part of the evaluation of patients on dialysis, in particular those with difficult BP control.

Blood Pressure Measurement in Dialysis Patients

Method of BP Measurement

Either auscultatory or oscillometric measurements are acceptable in dialysis patients [12]. As with any hypertensive patient, close attention to recommended guidelines for BP measurement is needed (e.g., the American Heart Association guidelines [13]), including avoidance of recent use of nicotine or caffeine. Because of the combined effects of aging and advanced kidney disease on arterial calcification, the possibility of noncompressibility of the brachial artery needs to be entertained as a cause of pseudohypertension. Patients should be screened by careful palpation of these vessels. Also, given the high prevalence of atherosclerotic peripheral arterial disease in ESKD, all patients should be screened periodically for inter-arm differences due to stenosis of the subclavian or axillary artery. If differences are observed, the arm with higher values should always be used. Unfortunately, performing this screen is problematic in HD patients with functional arteriovenous fistulae or grafts, which preclude BP measurement on their side. A means of bypassing this shortcoming is to check the BP in the thigh, using specific thigh cuffs. If the BP is higher in the thigh by >20 mmHg in the supine position, the patient should be monitored using the thigh, not the arm.

Orthostatic BP Measurement

Orthostatic hypotension (BP fall by >20/10 mmHg after 3 min of standing) is common in older patients, with or without a diagnosis of hypertension [14]. Among geriatric patients treated with antihypertensive drugs, orthostatic hypotension occurs in ~1/3 of patients. Patients on dialysis have impaired autonomic function and decreased baroreceptor sensitivity and are at increased risk for orthostatic hypotension. Furthermore, HD patients are at particularly increased risk of orthostasis following an HD session with ultrafiltration. All dialysis patients should have routine measurement of standing BP during all visits. HD patients must have standing BP measured prior to leaving the HD unit after a dialysis session.

"Location" of BP Measurement

There is growing evidence that the association between BP and outcomes is best assessed by BP measurements made outside of the office environment [1, 4, 10]. The most recent guidelines for patients with essential hypertension (2011 United Kingdom NICE guidelines and 2013 European Society of Hypertension guidelines) emphasize the importance of out-of-office BP monitoring for the diagnosis and management of hypertension. In dialysis patients, the observations are similar. Available cohort studies, although much smaller than in essential hypertension, corroborate the observations that out-of-office BP (48-h ambulatory BP or home BP) is a better predictor of mortality in HD patients. Data in PD are scarce but indicate greater ability of out-of-office BP to predict target organ damage (left ventricular hypertrophy, arterial stiffness) than conventional clinic BP measurements.

Besides the implications for prognosis, the following are relevant practical aspects of each type of monitoring:

- *Clinic (dialysis unit) BP*. This is by far the most applied in clinical practice, and it is the method adopted in the majority of studies that evaluated BP levels in maintenance HD. However, this method may be imprecise because HD facilities are very busy and BP measurements are usually not uniform and tend to overestimate BP compared with standardized measurements. Besides, in-center BP correlates poorly with interdialytic BP obtained by ambulatory BP monitoring. BP in peritoneal dialysis patients is more stable because PD patients do not have large variations in BP associated with fluid removal. Therefore, in PD patients BP can be better assessed by standard methods. When using clinic BP, it is important to make sure that devices are well calibrated, that cuff size matches the arm size of the patient, and that multiple readings are obtained and averaged. In HD patients, pre-, intra-, and post-HD values need to be integrated into the decision-making process (see below).
- *Home BP*. This is a simple and reliable method to estimate interdialytic BP profile and is superior to clinic BP as a guide to achieve BP control in HD patients. When performing home BP monitoring, patients should use a validated device (list available from www.dableducational.org) whose accuracy is confirmed by periodic matching with readings obtained by calibrated devices in the dialysis unit. Most guidelines recommend monitoring of BP twice a day (early in the morning before taking medications and in the evening before dinner) for a period of 5–7 days. If patients have symptoms suggestive of low BP, extra readings in the late morning and late evening can be added. We recommend that this monitoring be done once a month for HD patients and before every clinic visit for PD patients. Home systolic BP readings are typically 10/5 mmHg lower than office readings in the general population. In dialysis patients, however, the differences are smaller, typically less than 5 mmHg, possibly due to an underrepresentation of the white-coat effect and a higher prevalence of the "masked BP" effect in patients with advanced kidney disease.
- *Ambulatory BP monitoring (ABPM)*. ABPM is considered the gold standard in BP measurement in dialysis patients. In HD patients, ABPM shows the actual BP burden that occurs during the interdialytic period. ABPM also has better reproducibility as compared with clinic BP and is the only method that evaluates BP during sleep, which provides relevant prognostic data. However, the use ABPM in clinical practice is limited by operational difficulties (patients are often resistant to wearing the monitor during the interdialytic period), limited availability, and lack of reimbursement.

BP Profile in Dialysis Patients

The analysis of 44-h interdialytic ABPM in HD patients shows that even in patients who lower their BP during ultrafiltration, about 50 % returns to hypertensive levels within 12 h after HD [4]. Both awake and sleep BP increase between HD sessions, so that BP is higher in the second interdialytic day in comparison with the first interdialytic day. In patients dialyzed thrice weekly, the BP rise in the longer interdialytic period (72 h) in the third interdialytic day (measured by home BP) is attenuated in comparison with the first two interdialytic days.

The decrease in BP that normally happens during sleep is blunted in dialysis patients. Up to 80 % of HD patients are non-dippers (BP decrease less than 10 % during sleep), and a significant number of them are reverse dippers (BP higher during sleep). The possible causes of this abnormal circadian rhythm include volume overload, sleep-disordered breathing, and abnormalities in hormonal and neuroendocrine mediators mainly those associated with the sympathetic nervous system [4]. Non-dipping and reverse dipping may be associated with worse cardiovascular outcomes in dialysis patients. Due to fluctuations in cardiac output (intravascular volume changes) and increased arterial stiffness, systolic BP characteristically oscillates more than diastolic BP in dialysis patients, resulting in increased pulse pressure. No study has addressed BP profile specifically in the elderly dialysis patient.

BP Targets in Dialysis Patients

As noted above, many observational studies have shown an inverse relationship between BP and mortality in HD patients, whereas aggregate data from clinical trials actually suggest benefit from using antihypertensive agents in dialysis patients with hypertension. Reconciling these observations in the absence of definitive clinical trial data is difficult. Based on weak evidence, the Kidney Disease Outcome Quality Initiative (K/DOQI) guidelines recommended a target BP less than 140/90 mmHg pre-dialysis or less than 130/80 mmHg post-dialysis for HD patients [15]. These targets are reasonable, though one must understand that reaching these post-dialysis BP goals is associated with increased incidence of intradialytic hypotension.

One study compared the accuracy of the in-center BP measurements in conventional HD with interdialytic 44-h BP measured by ABPM, being considered hypertensive those patients with a 44-h average BP above 135/85 mmHg (levels extrapolated from the general population). In this study, pre-hemodialysis levels of 150/85 mmHg and post-hemodialysis levels of 130/75 mmHg had the best accuracy to diagnosis of interdialytic hypertension [16].

Overall, we do not disagree with the K/DOQI guidelines. However, we must be cognizant of the lack of data to support them. We find it more useful to use measures of interdialytic BP (home or ABPM) to assess overall BP control and to mitigate hypotension. As it relates to elderly patients, the situation is no different. However, given the evidence in the general population that elderly individuals may be at increased risk of worse outcomes when BP is lowered excessively, it may be prudent to use a more liberal approach to BP (i.e., higher BP targets, such as 150/90 mmHg) in elderly dialysis patients, particularly those aged 80 or older [17].

There are no specific guidelines for BP targets in PD patients; the K/DOQI guidelines do not provide any recommendations for this group of patients. We believe the practice should be similar to what is done in HD, using a clinic BP target of 140/90 mmHg in most patients (150/90 mmHg in older patients) [18].

Assessment of Target Organ Damage

We routinely evaluate target organ damage (heart, brain, large vessels, and eye) in dialysis patients. Patients should be routinely asked about symptoms related to these organs, including focal neurological deficits, symptoms of congestive heart failure, coronary disease, or peripheral arterial disease. Periodic examination of all patients should include a fundoscopic exam, with more detailed ophthalmologic evaluation in those with diabetes to identify the coexistence of retinal abnormalities. We obtain EKGs yearly, and all patients receive an echocardiogram to evaluate left ventricular mass and function, as these findings help guide treatment choices, such as the use of blockers of the renin-angiotensin system, vasodilating beta-blockers, and mineralocorticoid receptor antagonists in patients with systolic dysfunction.

Additionally, cardiovascular risk factor evaluation and modification is important, including advice about smoking cessation, increased aerobic exercise, evaluation and treatment of hyperlipidemia (preferably with a statin, although the clinical trial data in dialysis patients remain conflicting), and control of diabetes.

Management of Blood Pressure in Dialysis Patients

Knowledge of the multiple factors that can influence BP in dialysis patients (Table 7.1) and of disorders that are more prevalent in the elderly (Table 7.2) is important when making decisions regarding BP management in elderly dialysis patients. Mindful of these factors, the strategies to be used to control hypertension in dialysis involve four essential items: control of ECF volume through ultrafiltration, management of sodium balance through diet and dialysate prescription, judicious use of antihypertensive drugs, and consideration of alternative dialysis modalities, particularly daily and long-duration HD. Very limited data are specific to the elderly, so most of our recommendations listed below are based on data from the general dialysis population.

Table 7.2 Specific factors that can influence the management of blood pressure in elderly dialysis patients

Factor	Impact
Arterial stiffness	Difficult to control systolic BP
	Predisposition to intradialytic hypotension
Congestive heart failure	Dictates drug choices
	Predisposition to intradialytic hypotension
Cardiac arrhythmias	May dictate drug choices
Renovascular disease	Treatment may improve resistant hypertension (rare)
Thyroid disorders	If present, may increase BP. Screening and treatment is indicated
Sleep apnea (both obstructive and central)	Treatment with noninvasive positive-pressure ventilation improves BP

Control of Extracellular Fluid Volume

Sodium and water retention and their removal by the dialysis procedure have a pivotal role in determining BP levels and BP profile in dialysis patients. In dialysis patients with residual renal function, the use of diuretics can aid in the achievement of optimal volume control. The effective use of diuretics in dialysis patients often requires high oral doses of loop diuretics (e.g., furosemide 120–200 mg twice daily) in combination with a potent thiazide agent (e.g., metolazone 10 mg once or twice daily). This strategy could also avoid the need for aggressive ultrafiltration during dialysis.

In anuric dialysis patients, dietary sodium intake directly influences fluid ingestion and interdialytic weight gain [19]. This is because human physiology strives to preserve extracellular osmolality at an apparent fixed osmolar set point. In functionally anephric dialysis patients, the main osmolar regulator is thirst. For example, an HD patient who ingests 8 g of sodium chloride in one interdialytic day theoretically would have to ingest 1 l of water to maintain his or her osmolar homeostasis, and consequently, a small reduction of 2 g in sodium chloride ingestion a day may reduce 200 g in the daily weight gain. Thus, dietary sodium restriction, rather than fluid restriction, is critical in decreasing interdialytic weight gain and BP in HD patients. The same concept of an osmolar set point also determines the effect of dialysate sodium concentration on weight gain and BP. If the prescribed dialysate sodium concentration is higher than the patient's serum sodium concentration, then the high concentration gradient could result in unnecessary sodium load which in turn leads to fluid retention and hypertension [20]. Several studies in which the dialysate sodium prescription was reduced showed a reduction in interdialytic weight gain and BP. However, recent observational studies have raised concerns about the use of low dialysate sodium concentration [21]; therefore, large prospective studies will be necessary to guide the use of low dialysate sodium to control BP. It is safe to say, however, that high dialysate sodium or the use of sodium modeling should be avoided in hypertensive HD patients.

Assessment and Achievement of Dry Weight

The first step in BP control in HD patients is achieving the correct dry weight, which is the reference used in HD to determine the ultrafiltration volume in each HD session. In current clinical practice, dry weight is defined primarily as the weight at the end of the HD session that leaves the patient either without hypovolemia (hypotension and associated symptoms) or hypervolemia (hypertension or other evidence of volume overload). Although this approach seems reasonable, more specific estimations of extracellular volume have uncovered the inaccuracy of this clinical method [22, 23]. Bioimpedance analysis has shown that a large percentage (25–50 %) of patients have augmented ECF despite a normal clinical exam. Likewise, hypertensive HD patients who appear to be at their clinical dry weight often have a significant reduction in BP with a stepwise reduction (probing) of dry weight [9].

Figure 7.1 summarizes our proposed approach to the hypertensive dialysis patient who does not have obvious evidence of volume overload on clinical exam (pulmonary congestion, jugular venous distension, and edema). Assuming maximal dietary sodium restriction and limited sodium influx through the dialysate are already operative, we then proceed with increased ultrafiltration to lower the dry weight. In patients on conventional HD, we push the ultrafiltration targets by 0.3–0.5 kg per session so as to progressively lower the target post-HD weight. This is continued until the achievement of normotension or the development of intradialytic symptoms such as cramping, nausea/vomiting, chest pain, or intradialytic hypotension. In the elderly, dry weight accomplishment has to be cautious because older patients are at increased risk of intradialytic hypotension (see discussion below). Therefore, smaller increments in ultrafiltration targets are often indicated. In PD patients, increased ultrafiltration is achieved by increased PD fluid osmolality, or preferably, through the use of icodextrin, particularly in patients with peritoneal membrane with rapid solute transport characteristics.

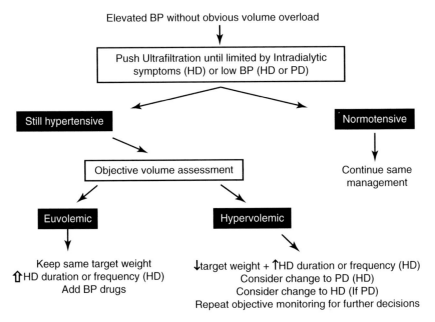

Fig. 7.1 Approach to blood pressure and volume management in dialysis patients. *BP* blood pressure, *HD* hemodialysis, *PD* peritoneal dialysis. Objective indicators of hypervolemia: inferior vena cava (IVC) ultrasound with inspiratory IVC collapse <25 %. Bioimpedance evidence of extracellular fluid volume excess (>25 % in women, >28 % in men). Blood volume (BV) monitoring evidence of flat residual BV slope (<1.33 %/h) during ultrafiltration. Can be used in hemodialysis patients only

If the patient remains hypertensive, objective assessment of ECF volume, if available, is indicated. The most accurate and best-studied method to determine ECF volume in dialysis patients is bioimpedance. The test provides a direct estimate of ECF volume with normative values for age and gender. A consensus position is that ECF volume expansion that is greater than 15 % of the predicted ECF volume is definitive evidence of volume overload. These measurements can be trended over time to evaluate the effectiveness of ultrafiltration. Inferior vena cava (IVC) ultrasound evaluates the changes in IVC diameter during the respiratory cycle as a marker of volume expansion. If the IVC diameter decreases by less than 25 % during inspiration, this is evidence of intravascular (and presumably ECF) volume expansion. Not as well studied but perhaps the most commonly available method to estimate ECF volume status is the analysis of blood volume changes during HD. Patients with ECF volume expansion have a flat slope of change in blood volume during ultrafiltration (less than 1.3 % per hour) [24]. As ultrafiltration rates are increased to achieve higher total ultrafiltration volumes, the slopes tend to change toward the target slope of 2.4–5.6 % per hour. When the slopes reach this range, there is no further benefit from ultrafiltration on BP reduction. For obvious reasons, blood volume monitoring cannot be used in PD patients.

After applying one of these objective measures of ECF volume expansion, we take the following approaches in case the patient remains hypertensive (Fig. 7.1):

1. In HD patients, if there is no evidence of ECF volume expansion, no further titration of dry weight is indicated. In such cases, the patient is declared resistant to pure control of ECF volume. There are two acceptable approaches to this problem: use of longer dialysis hours, use of short daily HD (e.g., 2 h/day 6 days/week), or addition of antihypertensive drugs. If it is a PD patient, the only possible resorts available are the use of drugs or conversion to long-hours HD or short daily HD. Because of issues regarding patient acceptance and lack of reimbursement for longer HD hours and/or increased HD frequency, these very effective options are largely underutilized in most countries, thus leading to the use of the second option, antihypertensive drugs (see below for details on their use).

2. If the patient remains hypertensive and the ECF volume is still expanded in an HD patient, dry weight needs to be titrated further down. The problem is that the reason why the dry weight could not be probed further was probably the development of intradialytic symptoms. In such case, the patient needs either a lower interdialytic weight gain to minimize ultrafiltration needs and improve HD tolerability or a slower means of volume removal, i.e., daily or long HD, or transfer to peritoneal dialysis.

3. By definition, patients who require objective measurement of ECF volume expansion cannot be adequately evaluated by the clinical exam. Therefore, if they remain hypertensive after changes outlined in #2, they require repeat objective assessment in order to delineate further treatment decisions.

Use of Antihypertensive Drugs in Elderly Dialysis Patients

Because of the limitations discussed above, drugs are often used to treat hypertension in the large majority of dialysis patients. As discussed before, two meta-analyses of randomized clinical trials have suggested cardiovascular and mortality benefit from antihypertensive drugs in dialysis patients. These trials included ACE inhibitors, angiotensin receptor blockers, calcium channel blockers, and the vasodilating beta-blocker carvedilol. More recent studies also suggest improved outcomes with the use of spironolactone [25, 26]. It is safe to say that most drug classes are effective in lowering BP in dialysis patients, with the exception of thiazides and loop diuretics in patients without residual renal function. In considering which drugs to use, we take into account the following elements:

1. Duration of action of the agent. Our preference is to use long-acting agents, as they make the treatment regimen easier for the patient. This is particularly important in elderly patients because of the frequent coexistence of cognitive impairment. In dialysis patients, the use of drugs that are excreted through the kidney is often preferable, as the absence of renal function increases their duration of action. For example, atenolol and lisinopril have been used with thrice weekly post-HD dosing in HD patients. This may be particularly useful in non-adherent patients, who can receive their medications immediately following HD under "directly observed therapy."
2. Removal of the agent by the dialysis procedure (relevant for HD patients). This has relevance to patients who have intradialytic hypertension (see below) and also to determine the need to provide any supplementation of agent following HD. Table 7.3 lists agents that are either not removed or only minimally removed by dialysis. It is important that the clinician becomes familiarized with the HD handling of the group of drugs that he/she preferentially uses in practice.
3. "Compelling" indications for a specific agent or drug class. This issue relates particularly to coexisting cardiovascular diseases (Table 7.4). Even though clinical trials in these conditions have rarely included dialysis patients, most experts agree that extrapolations from the general population are acceptable in the management of dialysis patients, thus guiding the choice of agent in many patients.
4. Potential relevance to problems commonly encountered in elderly patients. Table 7.5 lists clinical issues that are common in the elderly and that may call for a specific agent or drug class or may raise concerns about their use.

Table 7.3 Antihypertensive drugs that are not removed or only minimally removed by hemodialysis

ACE inhibitors	Benazepril, fosinopril
Angiotensin receptor blockers	Losartan, valsartan, telmisartan, candesartan
Calcium channel blockers	Amlodipine, felodipine, nifedipine, verapamil, diltiazem
α-blockers, β-blockers, and combined α- and β-blockers	Carvedilol, labetalol, bisoprolol, terazosin, doxazosin
Other agents	Clonidine, minoxidil

Table 7.4 Comorbid conditions that represent "compelling" indications for certain antihypertensive drug classes in hypertensive dialysis patients

Condition	Drug class(es) recommended
Heart failure with ↓ left ventricular systolic function	ACE inhibitors, angiotensin receptor blockers, vasodilating β-blockers, mineralocorticoid receptor antagonists
Coronary artery disease	β-blockers, ACE inhibitors
Left ventricular hypertrophy	Angiotensin receptor blockers, ACE inhibitors
Atrial fibrillation	β-blockers or non-DHP CCB (especially diltiazem) is the main agents used for heart rate control
Diabetes mellitus	ACE inhibitors or angiotensin receptor blockers
Stroke	ACE inhibitors (thiazides not indicated for this purpose in dialysis patients)

Table 7.5 Common clinical problems that may impact on antihypertensive drug choices in elderly dialysis patients

Condition	Comment
Cognitive dysfunction	Nonselective β-blockers (propranolol) and central antiadrenergic agents (clonidine, methyldopa) may rarely precipitate delirium
Depression	Lipophilic β-blockers (propranolol, metoprolol) may rarely increase depressive symptoms
High fall risk	Central antiadrenergics commonly cause excessive sedation and fatigue
Essential tremor	Nonselective β-blockers (propranolol) improve symptoms
Constipation (functional)	CCBs, especially non-DHP (diltiazem, verapamil), worsen colonic motility
Prostatic hyperplasia	α-blockers improve urine flow and obstructive voiding symptoms in dialysis patients who have residual urine output
Obstructive lung disease	β-blockers are generally safe, though may induce worsening symptoms in patients with significant airway reactivity

CCB calcium channel blocker, *DHP* dihydropyridines

Intradialytic Hypertension

The existence of patients who have an increase in BP during HD has long been recognized. However, recent cohort studies have described an association between an intradialytic rise in systolic BP (post-dialysis-pre-dialysis BP) of ≥10 mmHg and risk of death and hospitalization in HD patients. As a result, the increase in ≥10 mmHg has been used to define HD patients with intradialytic hypertension (ID-HTN), a process that occurs in 10–15 % of patients on conventional HD [10]. Interestingly, this definition includes patients who are normotensive at baseline, and in fact, one study showed that ID-HTN was associated with mortality only in patients with pre-HD SBP <120 mmHg. Patients with ID-HTN seem to be older and have lower body weight and evidence of undernutrition (lower serum creatinine and albumin levels). It thus appears that patients with ID-HTN may be sicker than patients who respond to UF with a fall in BP.

While not fully elucidated, the pathophysiology of ID-HTN is associated primarily with increased peripheral vascular resistance (Table 7.6). Faster plasma refilling

Table 7.6 Potential mechanisms associated with intradialytic hypertension

Patient factors:
Failure to reach estimated dry weight (i.e., volume overload)
Endothelial dysfunction:
HD removal of antihypertensive drugs
Hypokalemia
Dialysis procedure factors:
Dialysate composition (high sodium, high calcium, low potassium)

associated with volume overload could facilitate BP increase, and this hypothesis is corroborated by studies demonstrating less ID-HTN after aggressive probing of dry weight. Endothelial dysfunction resulting in increased vasoconstriction is characteristic of ID-HTN.

The management of ID-HTN requires a multipronged approach. First, one must ascertain that the patient is not volume expanded. If volume expanded, dry weight probing should take place as described above. In addition, factors such as high dialysate sodium and calcium must be avoided in the HD prescription, and prescribing antihypertensive drugs that are not removed in HD is a rational method in the treatment of ID-HTN. Finally, the vasodilating beta-blocker carvedilol, in doses of up to 50 mg twice daily, reduced the episodes of ID-HTN and improved endothelial function in a prospective crossover study of patients with ID-HTN [27].

Management of Intradialytic Hypotension in the Elderly

Unfortunately, the search for BP control in hypertensive HD patients often results in the dreaded complication of intradialytic hypotension (IDH), which is the fall in systolic BP by at least 20 mmHg accompanied by symptoms of organ ischemia that require intervention. IDH is the most common complication of HD, occurring in ~25 % of cases and in even higher rates among elderly patients and those with heart disease, diabetes, and autonomic neuropathy [10]. It is a consequence of an inadequate cardiovascular response to the reduction in blood volume during ultrafiltration. Because of impaired baroreflex function, elderly patients are particularly prone to IDH. Moreover, the consequences of IDH may be more severe in the elderly: dizziness, fatigue, and weakness may predispose to falls; underlying cerebrovascular disease may facilitate the occurrence of syncope, seizures, transient ischemic attacks, or stroke during IDH episodes; underlying coronary artery disease may result in myocardial infarction or cardiac arrhythmias during IDH; and repetitive episodes of IDH may be associated with asymptomatic myocardial ischemia and irreversible cardiac damage over time.

One or more of the factors that control BP in HD and keep hemodynamic stability can be affected in IDH-prone patients. Patient-specific factors and HD-related factors should be thought to prevent IDH episodes. These factors include aggressive ultrafiltration; decline in extracellular osmolality; impaired venoconstriction of the splanchnic circulation, which decreases venous pooling, impaired vascular response (decreased vasoconstriction or enhanced vasodilation); and structural heart disease. Identification of these processes is important in the mitigation of IDH.

Often in clinical practice, managing hypertension on the one hand and IDH on the other needs to take place. The management of IDH frequently requires multiple interventions that are summarized in Table 7.7. Finding the balance between BP control in the interdialytic period and BP "safety" during the HD session is a critical aspect of the care of complex elderly HD patients.

Table 7.7 Interventions for the management of intradialytic hypotension

Optimize dry weight, making sure that the patient is not volume depleted
Decrease interdialytic fluid gain
Treat reversible cardiac diseases (myocardial ischemia, aortic stenosis, pericardial effusion)
Adjust antihypertensive medications. Consider holding them on the days of HD. Consider evening dosing to minimize morning hypotension
High sodium dialysate or sodium modeling. Monitor interdialytic weight gain as it may increase
Ultrafiltration profiling (often combined with sodium modeling). Consider longer HD or addition of extra sessions to avoid the use of fast ultrafiltration rates
Avoid food during dialysis
Cool dialysate (~36° Celsius)
Avoid low-calcium dialysate
Correct severe anemia
Screen for and correct carnitine deficiency if present
Pharmacological therapy: midodrine (2.5–15 mg orally given 15 min prior to HD)

Key Points
1. Orthostatic hypotension is common in the elderly. HD patients must have standing BP measured prior to leaving the HD unit after a dialysis session.
2. Extracellular volume overload is the most important reason for hypertension in elderly dialysis patients.
3. Achievement of dry weight must be cautious in the elderly dialysis patient.
4. Choice of antihypertensive drugs often depends on comorbid conditions that are common in the elderly.
5. Intradialytic hypotension and intradialytic hypertension are adverse intradialytic events that are more frequent in the elderly.
6. Longer HD hours and short daily HD should be considered for a better BP control in the elderly dialysis patients.

References

1. Agarwal R (2012) The controversies of diagnosing and treating hypertension among hemodialysis patients. Semin Dial 25:370–376
2. Ortega LM, Materson BJ (2011) Hypertension in peritoneal dialysis patients: epidemiology, pathogenesis, and treatment. J Am Soc Hypertens 5:128–136
3. Myers OB, Adams C, Rohrscheib MR et al (2010) Age, race, diabetes, blood pressure, and mortality among hemodialysis patients. J Am Soc Nephrol 21:1970–1978
4. Peixoto AJ, Santos SF (2010) Blood pressure management in hemodialysis: what have we learned? Curr Opin Nephrol Hypertens 19:561–566
5. Zoccali C (2003) Arterial pressure components and cardiovascular risk in end-stage renal disease. Nephrol Dial Transplant 18:249–252
6. Agarwal R, Sinha AD (2009) Cardiovascular protection with antihypertensive drugs in dialysis patients: systematic review and meta-analysis. Hypertension 53:860–866
7. Heerspink HJ, Ninomiya T, Zoungas S, de Zeeuw ZD, Grobbee DE, Jardine MJ, Gallagher M, Roberts MA, Cass A, Neal B, Perkovic V (2009) Effect of lowering blood pressure on cardiovascular events and mortality in patients on dialysis: a systematic review and meta-analysis of randomised controlled trials. Lancet 373:1009–1015
8. Laegreid I, Bye A, Asarod K, Jordhoy M (2012) Nutritional problems, overhydration and the association with quality of life in elderly dialysis patients. Int Urol Nephrol 44:1185–1192
9. Agarwal R, Alborzi P, Satyan S, Light RP (2009) Dry-weight reduction in hypertensive hemodialysis patients (DRIP): a randomized, controlled trial. Hypertension 53:500–507
10. Santos SF, Peixoto AJ, Perazella MA (2012) How should we manage adverse intradialytic blood pressure changes? Adv Chronic Kidney Dis 19:158–165
11. Briet M, Boutouyrie P, Laurent S, London GM (2012) Arterial stiffness and pulse pressure in CKD and ESRD. Kidney Int 82:388–400
12. Sankaranarayanan N, Santos SFF, Peixoto AJ (2004) Blood pressure measurement in dialysis patients. Adv Chron Kidney Dis 11:134–142
13. Pickering TG, Hall JE, Appel LJ et al (2005) Recommendations for blood pressure measurement in humans and experimental animals. Part 1: blood pressure measurement in humans: a statement for professionals from the subcommittee of professional and public education of the american heart association council on high blood pressure research. Hypertension 45:142–161
14. Reddy AK, Jogendra M, Rosendorff C (2014) Blood pressure measurement in the geriatric population. Blood Press Monit 19:59–63
15. K/DOQI Clinical Practice Guidelines for Cardiovascular Disease in Dialysis Patients (2005) Blood pressure. Am J Kidney Dis 45(Suppl 3):S49–S57
16. Agarwal R, Lewis R (2001) Prediction of hypertension in chronic hemodialysis patients. Kidney Int 60:1982–1989
17. James PA, Oparil S, Carter BL et al (2014) 2014 evidence-based guideline for the management of high blood pressure in adults report from the panel members appointed to the eighth joint national committee (JNC 8). JAMA 311:507–520
18. Aronow WS, Fleg JL, Pepine CJ, Artinian NT et al (2011) ACCF/AHA 2011 expert consensus document on hypertension in the elderly: a report of the American College of Cardiology Foundation Task Force on Clinical Expert Consensus. J Am Soc Hypertens 5:259–352
19. Santos SFF, Peixoto AJ (2010) Sodium balance in maintenance hemodialysis. Semin Dial 23:549–555
20. Santos SF, Peixoto AJ (2008) Revisiting the dialysate sodium prescription as a tool for better blood pressure and interdialytic weight gain management in hemodialysis patients. Clin J Am Soc Nephrol 3:522–530
21. Hecking M, Karaboyas A, Saran R et al (2012) Dialysate sodium concentration and the association with interdialytic weight gain, hospitalization and mortality. Clin J Am Soc Nephrol 7:92–100

22. Dou Y, Zhu F, Kotanko P (2012) Assessment of extracellular fluid volume and fluid status in hemodialysis patients: current status and technical advances. Semin Dial 25:377–387
23. Levin NW, Kotanko P, Eckardt KU, Kasiske BL, Chazot C, Cheung AK, Redon J, Wheeler DC, Zoccali C, London GM (2010) Blood pressure in chronic kidney disease stage 5D-report from a kidney disease: improving global outcomes controversies conference. Kidney Int 77:273–284
24. Sinha AD, Light LP, Agarwal R (2010) Relative plasma volume monitoring during hemodialysis aids the assessment of dry weight. Hypertension 55:305–311
25. Matsumoto Y, Mori Y, Kageyama S et al (2014) Spironolactone reduces cardiovascular and cerebrovascular morbidity and mortality in hemodialysis patients. J Am Coll Cardiol 63:528–536
26. Ito Y, Mizuno M, Suzuki Y et al (2014) Long term effects of spironolactone in peritoneal dialysis patients. J Am Soc Nephrol 25:1094–1102
27. Inrig JK, Van Buren P, Kim C, Vongpatanasin W, Povsic TJ, Toto R (2012) Probing the mechanisms of intradialytic hypertension: a pilot study targeting endothelial cell dysfunction. Clin J Am Soc Nephrol 7:1300–1309

Chapter 8
A Sensible Approach to Address Dialysis Adequacy in the Elderly

Nicole Stankus and John T. Daugirdas

Introduction

A number of relevant issues regarding whether to start dialysis or manage an older patient with conservative therapy and whether to start hemodialysis or peritoneal dialysis are covered in other chapters of this handbook. This chapter is limited to the question of what sort of hemodialysis or peritoneal dialysis prescription we should write for an older patient, once the decision has been made to manage their advanced symptomatic kidney disease with chronic renal replacement therapy.

Hemodialysis

With regard to hemodialysis prescription, the following questions can be asked:

1. *Should greater use of twice-weekly dialysis be recommended for some older patients?*
2. *Is a minimum single-pool Kt/V of 1.2 as recommended by KDOQI [1] or ~1.35 as recommended by the European Best Practices Group (EBPG) [2] appropriate for older patients?*
3. *Should the minimum session length be 3 h as recommended by KDOQI, or 4 h as recommended by the ERBPG? Should there be a maximum ultrafiltration rate of 10–13 ml/kg/h?*
4. *Should high-flux membranes be used routinely? Is there a benefit to hemodiafiltration?*

N. Stankus, MD (✉) • J.T. Daugirdas, MD
Department of Nephrology, University of Illinois at Chicago,
Chicago, IL, USA
e-mail: nstankus@medicine.bsd.uchicago.edu; jtdaugir@uic.edu

© Springer Science+Business Media New York 2016
M. Misra (ed.), *Dialysis in Older Adults: A Clinical Handbook*,
DOI 10.1007/978-1-4939-3320-4_8

5. *Should home hemodialysis, in-center nocturnal dialysis, and more frequent dialysis be utilized more frequently in the older adults? Is it possible to overdialyze older patients?*
6. *Is there a role for a palliative dialysis only to control symptoms of uremia and volume overload?*

Quality of evidence

It should be pointed out that in the area of adequacy for both hemodialysis and peritoneal dialysis, high-level evidence in the form of randomized trials simply does not exist. The basic recommendation for a minimum Kt/V of 1.2 in hemodialysis patients stems from the National Cooperative Dialysis Study, where Kt/V was a secondary analysis [3], and the NIH HEMO Trial, which failed to find a benefit of higher doses of dialysis [4]. Data from the European NECOSAD group suggest that when substantial residual kidney function is present, the dose of dialysis given has little effect on outcomes, and the 2006 KDOQI adequacy guidelines were written to apply to patients with residual kidney clearance of urea <2 ml/min/1.73 m^2.

As opposed to randomized trials, a large number of observational datasets exist, suggesting optimum or minimum doses of either hemodialysis or peritoneal dialysis. However, analysis of such results is complicated by the occurrence of "dose-targeting bias," where patients achieving a certain dose target appear to have better survival that is not related to the biological effects of dose. This dose-targeting bias can result in an apparent never-ending increase in an apparent minimum dose of dialysis, as dose targets are progressively raised. Dose-targeting bias can also result in artifactual "benefits" of extending dialysis time beyond a certain target, such as 4 h, where very marked apparent improvement is seen with only trivially longer dialysis sessions when sessions above and below a given target are compared [5].

Older patients form a heterogeneous group with strikingly different levels of physical and cognitive function and goals of care. First of all, there are patients in the 65–80 year range, which were included in many of the trials used to establish dialysis dose targets, and then there are patients older than 80 years, who were excluded from most trials. Some older patients may be frail, have marked cognitive impairment, and be on the border of being best treated by dialysis vs. by some form of nondialysis palliative care, whereas there is a subset of healthy older people who have survived intact to a sometimes a very old age who have activity and independence levels typically found only in much younger patients. Frailty is commonly seen in older adults not only for reasons related to uremia but to lack of financial or social support or because of comorbidities. It is usually very easy to reach conventional adequacy targets in malnourished patients, because their body size is quite small, and both hemodialysis and peritoneal dialysis guideline groups sometimes recommend dialysis targets based on median standard body weight based on height, weight, age, and frame size as opposed to current weight. Then there is another subgroup of markedly obese older patients, in whom it may be difficult to deliver conventional adequacy targets due to their relatively high total body water volume.

Perhaps the minimum amount of small molecular weight solute clearance prescribed during dialysis should be a certain minimum percentage of the GFR found normally in healthy age and sex-matched controls. Median GFR does decrease as we age, but it is not clear whether this is a physiological change, reflecting sufficiency of a lower GFR, or progressive loss of renal reserve. In the latter instance, the minimum solute clearance should theoretically be unchanged.

Aging is associated with many changes in body composition. As a rule, percent body fat increases and lean mass and bone mineral density and fat-free mass (FFM) decrease. Body composition changes associated with aging often occur in the absence of weight fluctuations. In the Fels Longitudinal Study, from 18 to 64 years of age, TBW volume for men did not decline with age, and the age-related decrease of TBW in women was small [6]. Bioimpedance studies in healthy well-hydrated older adults also showed that TBW was not significantly different, FFM is significantly lower, and FFM hydration ratio (TBW/FFM) is higher than in the younger adults [7]. However, lean body mass and TBW decrements occur in subjects older than 70. Many older patients tend to be small, and their ratio of TBW/BSA will be low. A surface-area scaled approach to dosing dialysis would suggest that in such patients with a low TBW/BSA ratio, the recommended minimum spKt/V values of 1.2 or even 1.4 according to European standards, might not be adequate.

According to DOPPS findings, hemodialysis prescription and clinical practices in older patients mainly reflected country-specific practices [8]. Mean prescribed blood flow rate was virtually identical in all age groups in most countries, between 295 and 395 ml/min, except for Japan, which displayed a mean blood flow rate between 184 and 207 ml/min. The mean duration of dialysis sessions was about 15 min shorter in older than in younger patients across various regions of the world. However, once the prescribed treatment time was normalized for body weight, no significant differences were observed across age groups. No differences were observed in the delivered dialysis dose, as measured by single-pool *Kt/V*, which was similar in all age categories within each region. Maintenance of a satisfactory dialysis dose can be partially explained by the lower dry weight and lower lean body mass, which were common in the older group. The mean ultrafiltration rate was lower in the older than in the younger age groups. This is likely explained by a lower sodium intake.

1. *Should greater use of twice-weekly dialysis be recommended for some older patients?*

Twice-a-week dialysis has generally been frowned upon as a therapy option. Theoretical analyses of equivalent weekly clearances such as standard Kt/V suggest that in the absence of residual kidney function, it is difficult to reach the currently recommended minimum standard Kt/V value of 2.0 or 2.15 (the minimum value depends on what method is used to calculate standard Kt/V). In patients dialyzed three times per week, there also is the issue of increased mortality that seems to occur on Monday or Tuesday, i.e., after the long interdialytic interval. With a twice-weekly dialysis schedule, every interval is "long"; in fact, one interval is "long," comparable to the weekend interval with a 3/week schedule, and the other is "very long," being 1 day greater. Nevertheless, in a rather large cross-sectional US study, twice-a-week dialysis was associated with slightly better outcome instead of the expected results (worse outcome) [9]. This result was likely due to patient selection. Recent data from China has shown similar survival in patients dialyzed 2/week and 3/week. [10]; plus incident patients with substantial residual renal function who begin dialysis using a 2/week schedule appear to have a slower rate of loss of urine output.

These findings suggest that perhaps while twice-a-week schedules should be prescribed only in unusual circumstances in anuric patients of any age, that usage of such a schedule could be liberalized in older patients with substantial residual urine volume. In this regard, CMS quality measures need to carefully mirror the thoughtful 2006 KDOQI guidelines, which did not disallow twice-a-week schedules for patients with residual urea clearances greater than 2 ml/min per 1.73 m².

2. *Is a minimum single-pool Kt/V of 1.2 as recommended by KDOQI or ~1.35 as recommended by the European Best Practices Group (EBPG) appropriate for older patients?*

Although the very older were excluded from the NCDS study, cross-sectional data, which often does include older subjects, suggest an exponential rise in mortality as Kt/V decreases to very low values. When one starts to get below a Kt/V of 0.9, even short-term outcomes deteriorate. For the general dialysis population as a whole, these minimum Kt/V values are being far exceeded, especially in smaller patients. Again, KDOQI 2006 limits these guidelines to patients with minimum degrees of residual kidney function, basing the recommendation of the data from NECOSAD [11].

For anuric older patients and especially older women who are small in size, due to either malnutrition or because they always were small, the question might be whether to increase the amount of dialysis based on body surface-area considerations. The answer to this question is not known and is purely opinion based. Guidelines suggest giving more dialysis to poorly nourished subjects, with the hope of increasing appetite, but while this might work in the Kt/V range below 1.2, in the HEMO study, there was no apparent nutrition benefit of moving from a Kt/V of 1.3 to about 1.7. Similarly, in the Frequent Hemodialysis Network (FHN) trial, providing very large increments in the standard Kt/V in terms of 6/week daily or nocturnal dialysis did not result in any improvement in lean body weight or serum albumin [12]. Conversely, if there is difficulty in achieving a Kt/V > 1.2 in a very large patient, surface-area considerations suggest that one might be able to dialyze such a patient with a slightly lower Kt/V, while giving a surface-area-adjusted dose of dialysis that would be similar to a dose > 1.2 in an average-sized patient.

3. *Should the minimum session length be 3 h as recommended by KDOQI or 4 h as recommended by the ERBPG? Should maximum ultrafiltration rate be limited to 10–13 ml/kg/h?*

There is an increasing tendency by guideline and regulatory groups to set a minimum dialysis session length as a quality target. Currently KDOQI as a clinical practice recommendation suggests a minimum time of 3 h for patients with minimal residual kidney function, while the EBPG recommends 4 h. Weekly dialysis time affects removal of molecules such as phosphorus as well as middle molecules, the concentration of which does not progressively decrease to a great extent during a dialysis session and especially those solutes which maintain relatively high plasma concentrations after the first 3 h of a dialysis session. Weekly dialysis time also affects ultrafiltration rate. Ultrafiltration rate depends completely on three variables: weekly fluid ingestion, weekly urine output, and weekly dialysis time. In the USA, the median value is close to 10 mL/kg/h, and various studies have suggested worse outcomes when the UF rate exceeds 10 or in some studies, 12–13 ml/kg/h. A recent abstract suggested that sizing target UF rate per kg body weight is not an optimum approach, as it resulted in different risk profiles for small and large patients and for men and women; a more consistent risk profile was obtained by a cutoff of 800 ml/h (Lacson-JR et al., ASN abstract, JASN Sep. 2014) regardless of body size.

The data for session length beyond 3.5 h affecting outcome are very much country dependent, and in the USA, in some studies, there is no apparent benefit. There may to be a dose-targeting bias effect, as in those countries where 4 h is targeted, e.g., Japan, the session length appears to affect mortality to an especially great extent [5].

Older patients often are more compliant with dietary restrictions than their younger counterparts. They eat less sodium and also less meat, which should lower their phosphorus intake. Thus, even anuric older may achieve Kt/V targets with session lengths substantially lower than 4 h. In older patients with substantial urine output, even a minimum treatment time of 3 h may be unnecessary if interdialytic weight gain is modest and ultrafiltration is well tolerated.

4. *Should high-flux membranes or hemodiafiltration be used routinely in the older?*

Recent meta-analyses of controlled studies suggest that the main benefit of using of high-flux dialysis is a modest reduction in terms of cardiovascular mortality. No benefit in terms of quality of life, anemia control, or nutrition was seen in these studies, and in those studies which identified prespecified subgroups, age was not one of the subgroups that had particular benefit from removal of middle molecules. In particular, the large "CONTRAST" study, which compared hemodiafiltration with low-flux hemodialysis, failed to show a benefit in overall survival or in cardiac structure [13]. Over time, there was a slight lowering of inflammatory mediators, but this was apparent only after 2 years of treatment. All in all, these data argue that any benefits of high-flux dialysis or hemodiafiltration in the older adults would be modest. If high-flux dialyzer membranes or HDF are being used routinely, there is no reason not to use them in the older, but there should be no expectation that an older dialysis patient would be having any particularly benefit.

5. *Should home hemodialysis, in-center nocturnal dialysis, and more frequent dialysis be utilized more frequently in the older adults? Is it possible to overdialyze older patients?*

There appears to be a marked survival advantage in patients being dialyzed at home compared to those being dialyzed in-center, even when comparable doses of dialysis are being given. Although this has been ascribed completely to patient selection (more motivated, self-actuated patients with greater family and social support structure having better survival), there may be real advantages to home hemodialysis, including less exposure to infectious agents, less interruption of meals, and increased time for work and hobbies. On the other hand, in some older patients with limited social and family support, especially those living alone, in-center dialysis may provide an appreciated and needed source of social interaction.

In terms of more frequent dialysis, in the FHN and other trials, it has been shown that a more frequent "daily" (5–6 times/week) schedule improves left ventricular hypertrophy and physical functioning and also resulted in slightly improved control of phosphorus, a substantial decrease in the need blood pressure medications, and a significant reduction in blood pressure. In other studies, frequent dialysis has been associated with reduced myocardial stunning and post-dialysis recovery time. More recently matched cohort data suggest that relative to thrice-weekly in-center hemodialysis, daily home hemodialysis associates with modest improvements in survival. However, benefits from frequent home hemodialysis on mortality in the older patients maybe be reduced and significant support from a caregiver may be needed to overcome age-related physical and mental limitations.

Some patients do complain of feeling "overdialyzed," and this can appear with long session lengths given 3 times per week, as well as with frequent long nocturnal dialysis. It is unclear to what extent these symptoms may be due to excessive ECF volume reduction or to removal of some as yet undefined solute. To date, no one has identified key substances which may be excessively removed from the blood during dialysis, apart from certain vitamins. In fact, in high-flux dialysis, vitamin B12 supplementation has been shown to reduce ESA requirements. B12 deficiency is common in the older adults, many of whom are on proton pump inhibitors. An additional depletion that is known to occur with long and frequent dialysis is that of phosphorus, and this may be particularly important in older patients who follow a diet relatively low in phosphorus, as well as potassium, and depletion can occur in the very older who are not ingesting an adequate diet, even with more conventional dialysis schedules.

6. *In older patients on the border between dialysis care and palliative care, can dialysis be given in a palliative fashion to control any distressing symptoms?*

Kidney transplantation reduces mortality compared to staying on dialysis in all ages; however, surgery itself temporarily increases the risk of death. Therefore, the mortality benefits associated with kidney transplantation (regardless of donor type) are restricted to older patients with reasonable baseline life expectancy and without dramatically increased perioperative risk. The majority of older patients on RRT thus are on dialysis for the rest of their life. UK Renal Registry 2012 data show that median survival for patients >75 years old is only 2.4 years. For frail patients, survival rates are considerably worse and often accompanied by a marked decline in physical function. A recent Canadian longitudinal study of 97 patients >80 years old showed a dramatic reduction in physical function within the first 6 months of starting dialysis [14]. At the start, 75 % of patients were functionally independent and living at home; by 6 months, a further 30 % required community support or transfer to a nursing home. At 12 months, only 22 % remained alive and independent.

In patients who are deteriorating slowly, the question of ceasing dialysis abruptly vs. reducing the amount of dialysis to control most pressing symptoms can arise.

For example, such patients may be eating small amounts of food, with little difficulty in control of phosphorus, potassium, or ECF due to low intake of phosphorus and sodium. Alkalosis is prevalent in patients eating limited amounts of protein. Thus, it may be reasonable to reduce the amount of dialysis in such patients to a level needed to control volume and potassium, phosphorus, and bicarbonate, until a decision can be reached to change to completly palliative care.

Peritoneal Dialysis Adequacy, Age, and Outcomes

With regard to peritoneal dialysis, the questions might be:

1. *Should the general guideline for a minimum weekly Kt/V of 1.7 be maintained in the older?*
2. *Is there any advantage of APD over CAPD in terms of adequacy in this patient group?*

General Issues Regarding PD Versus HD in the Older Adults

Choice of PD over HD is a complex one and influenced heavily by physicians' targeting improved long-term survival on RRT. Age plays a significant role in dialysis mortality. The debate on whether PD is equally beneficial in younger vs. older patient with and without serious comorbidities has been going on due to disparate outcomes of various studies. Earlier studies indicated that PD was more beneficial in younger patients (<60–65 years old) without comorbidities, while HD was more beneficial in older patients. Superiority of HD in diabetics over the age of 45 with or without other comorbidities has been shown, summarizing the rather widely accepted view that being older and having multiple comorbid conditions favor better outcomes with HD. However, patients on PD, both incident and prevalent, historically tended to be younger; thus, adjustment for age is essential when comparing mortality data. Importantly, most studies agreed that risk of death is generally lower on PD during first 2 years of dialysis.

Recently, the focus of discussion has shifted from the survival on RRT to the quality of life (QoL), especially in older adults where emphasis is shifting to the age-appropriate care. For the fit older patient, PD enables individuals to travel and have an active social life. The frail older often tolerate HD poorly because of hemodynamic instability and require transportation to and from dialysis. PD can help with these difficulties.

Assisted PD is a proven way to increase the overall number of older patients who can be treated with PD at home despite having very severe comorbidities.

In nursing homes, assisted PD allows the patient's daytime to be used for other activities and enables better rehabilitation. Also, in the USA, a new trend of "home hemodialysis" has established itself in nursing homes, when patients receive 3 h of low-efficiency dialysis 5–6 days a week.

1. *Should the general guideline for a minimum weekly Kt/V of 1.7 be maintained in the older patients?*

The original recommendation for a weekly Kt/V of 2.1 in PD was based on results of the CANUSA study; however, it later became apparent that the benefits of higher dialysis dose were limited to that component of dose provided by residual kidney function [15]. The ADEMEX trial then showed that results were no poorer in patients being dialyzed to a weekly Kt/V of 1.7, and that is where we stand today. In peritoneal dialysis, as dose of dialysis is decreased, the level of peritoneal clearance at which outcomes begin to deteriorate simply is not known. Which V to use for calculating Kt/V is an issue in PD: V from standard weights obtained from NHANES results in a targets for Kt/V adjusted for obese and for thin and frail patients. Under current guidelines, a weekly Kt/V of 1.7 is recommended regardless of whether a dry day or continuous modality of PD is used, and weekly creatinine clearance is relegated to a subsidiary role.

There is no special evidence suggesting that a dose of PD lower than 1.7 might be acceptable in the older patient, but on the other hand, there is little evidence to suggest that lowering the dose below this value is of harm in general. In PD the dose is calculated as the sum of residual renal and peritoneal clearances, and the extent of residual kidney function is of key importance in maintaining good outcome. Once residual kidney function is lost, then peritoneal clearance obviously becomes the foundation of PD, but even then, there is little formal evidence that, for example, anuric PD patients treated with a weekly Kt/V of 1.4 have increased risk of adverse events relative to those receiving weekly Kt/V values that meet or exceed the current target of 1.7. By choosing PD in older adults, we emphasize that QoL and age-appropriate interventions are preferred to the more aggressive approaches that may insignificantly prolong life. Because the adequacy data for PD are so limited, one should apply clinical judgment and use guideline-recommended Kt/V targets with discretion. In many cases, a Kt/V of 1.5 with sustainable peritoneal prescription is more beneficial to a frail, older patient than a prescription delivering a higher Kt/V that requires an onerous schedule and that might lead to patient and caregiver burnout.

APD with a dry day, in combination with some degree of residual renal function, may allow attainment of target weekly Kt/V in frail older patients. Care should be exercised when introducing icodextrin solutions to the PD prescription, as it may produce excessive ultrafiltration in the very frail and result in volume depletion and hypotension. It should be remembered that ultrafiltration in PD is magnified in patients with low serum albumin due to reduced plasma oncotic pressure, a caveat that applies to patients of any age group.

2. *Is there any advantage of APD over CAPD in terms of adequacy in this patient group?*

In earlier iterations of dosing guidelines for PD, the recommended weekly Kt/V urea dose was higher for APD than for CAPD, and a second dosing target based on weekly creatinine clearance was designed to focus on removal of larger weight molecules which equilibrate relatively slowly with peritoneal dialysate. Currently,

PD is often given as a blend of APD and CAPD, using APD at night and one or two exchanges during the day as needed to control fluid. The increased practicality of treating older patients with APD discussed above, combined with poorer tolerance of daytime fills, makes APD the therapy of choice for the majority of older patients.

Summary

In deciding an appropriate dose of dialysis for older patients, flexibility is the key, and the relative lack of high-level evidence behind current "quality" adequacy guidelines needs to be kept in mind. The dose of dialysis needs to be individualized, and in patients with significant urine output, dose can be reduced from that recommended by guidelines that were designed primarily for patients with little residual renal function.

Modern dialysis care should focus on alleviating bothersome symptoms and enabling patients to achieve their goals for living.

Key Points

1. Aging is associated with many changes in body composition: percent of body fat increases, lean mass and bone mineral density and fat-free mass decrease, and total body water essentially stays stable. Thus, a physiologic rationale to alter the HD dose in the older is not clear, except in small patients with a low TBW/BSA ratio, where a surface-area-scaled approach to dosing dialysis would suggest prescribing higher than the minimum spKt/V.

2. On a thrice-weekly schedule, a minimum treatment time of 3 h may be unnecessary if interdialytic weight gain is modest and ultrafiltration is well tolerated. Twice-a-week HD schedules could be used in older patients with substantial residual urine volume or in patients who are transitioning to complete palliative care.

3. Benefits of high-flux dialysis or hemodiafiltration would be modest; the impact on mortality of daily home hemodialysis would be lower in the older adults, and selection of home vs. in-center dialysis should be made base on patient preference and availability of appropriate family and social support.

4. When prescribing PD, the prescription should be written to maximize non-intrusiveness of the therapy. Usually, this means greater use of APD and APD with a dry day in particular. The target weekly Kt/V prescription should be set according to clinical judgment, seeking to maximize technique survival and patient comfort.

References

1. National Kidney Foundation (2006) KDOQI clinical practice guideline and clinical practice recommendations: hemodialysis adequacy, peritoneal dialysis adequacy, and vascular access: update 2006. Am J Kidney Dis 48(suppl 1):S1–S322
2. European Best Practice Guidelines Expert Group on Hemodialysis ErRA (2002) Section II. Haemodialysis adequacy. Nephrol Dial Transplant 17(Suppl 7):16–31
3. Lowrie EG, Laird NM, Parker TF et al (1981) Effect of the hemodialysis prescription of patient morbidity: report from the National Cooperative Dialysis Study. N Engl J Med 305:1176–1181
4. Moret KE, Grootendorst DC, Dekker FW et al (2012) Agreement between different parameters of dialysis dose in achieving treatment targets: results from the NECOSAD study. Nephrol Dial Transplant 27:1145–1152
5. Daugirdas JT (2013) Dialysis time, survival, and dose-targeting bias. Kidney Int 83:9–13
6. Chumlea WC, Guo SS, Zeller CM et al (1999) Total body water data for white adults 18 to 64 years of age: the Fels Longitudinal Study. Kidney Int 56:244–252
7. Buffa R, Floris GU, Putzu PF et al (2011) Body composition variations in ageing. Coll Antropol 35:259–265
8. Canaud B, Tong L, Tentori F et al (2011) Clinical practices and outcomes in elderly hemodialysis patients: results from the Dialysis Outcomes and Practice Patterns Study (DOPPS). Clin J Am Soc Nephrol 6:1651–1662
9. Hanson JA, Hulbert-Shearon TE, Ojo AO et al (1999) Prescription of twice-weekly hemodialysis in the USA. Am J Nephrol 19:625–633
10. Bieber B, Qian J, Anand S et al (2014) Two-times weekly hemodialysis in China: frequency, associated patient and treatment characteristics and Quality of Life in the China Dialysis Outcomes and Practice Patterns study. Nephrol Dial Transplant 29:1770–1777
11. Merkus MP, Jager KJ, Dekker FW et al (2000) Predictors of poor outcome in chronic dialysis patients: The Netherlands Cooperative Study on the Adequacy of Dialysis. The NECOSAD Study Group. Am J Kidney Dis 35:69–79
12. Chertow GM, Levin NW, Beck GJ et al (2010) In-center hemodialysis six times per week versus three times per week. N Engl J Med 363:2287–2300
13. Grooteman MP, van den Dorpel MA, Bots ML et al (2012) Effect of online hemodiafiltration on all-cause mortality and cardiovascular outcomes. J Am Soc Nephrol 23:1087–1096
14. Jassal SV, Chiu E, Hladunewich M (2009) Loss of independence in patients starting dialysis at 80 years of age or older. N Engl J Med 361:1612–1613
15. Adequacy of dialysis and nutrition in continuous peritoneal dialysis: association with clinical outcomes. Canada-USA (CANUSA) Peritoneal Dialysis Study Group (1996) J Am Soc Nephrol 7:198–207

Chapter 9
Anemia Management in the Elderly Dialysis Patient: Is It Different?

Iain C. Macdougall

Introduction

Prior to the 1990s, anemia management in the dialysis patient was fairly limited and was clearly suboptimal. Several strategies were tested and occasionally implemented, including iron supplementation and replacement of other hematinics, such as vitamin B_{12} or folic acid, and the use of androgens (which are weak stimulators of erythropoiesis). Many dialysis patients remained severely anemic and were supported by regular red cell transfusions, which often had to be administered every 2–4 weeks to patients whose baseline hemoglobin concentration was about 5 or 6 g/dL. Transient increases in the hemoglobin concentration to levels of around 10 or 11 g/dL were seen following the blood transfusions, but within a few weeks, the hemoglobin concentration had once again fallen to the baseline level of around 5–6 g/dL. Further transfusions were administered, and this desperate cycle of treatment repeated itself, resulting in transfusional iron overload. Thus, it was not uncommon for dialysis patients to run serum ferritin concentrations in the 1000's. Other complications of blood transfusions included the transmission of infectious agents, particularly viral, as well as transfusion reactions, including transfusion-related acute lung injury (TRALI) and transfusion-associated circulatory overload (TACO). Although rare, such complications could be devastating. Another important complication of blood transfusions includes HLA sensitization, which renders subsequent renal transplantation problematic; although this remains a concern, it is clearly of little relevance to elderly dialysis patients, most of whom are not suitable for kidney transplantation.

The original version of this chapter was revised.
An erratum to this chapter can be found at DOI 10.1007/978-1-4939-3320-4_17

I.C. Macdougall, BSc, MD, FRCP
Department of Renal Medicine, King's College Hospital, London, UK

Renal Unit, King's College Hospital, London SE5 9RS, UK
e-mail: iain.macdougall@nhs.net

© Springer Science+Business Media New York 2016
M. Misra (ed.), *Dialysis in Older Adults: A Clinical Handbook*,
DOI 10.1007/978-1-4939-3320-4_9

The advent of recombinant human erythropoietin in the late 1980s heralded a logical and much more satisfactory solution to the management of anemia in dialysis patients [1, 2]. For the first time, it was possible to achieve a steady and sustained increase in hemoglobin concentration without transfusional support, and indeed the use of red cell transfusions in hemodialysis patients dramatically decreased during the 1990s. Recombinant human erythropoietin or epoetin, as it became known, was followed by two other erythropoietic agents, namely, darbepoetin alfa and pegylated epoetin beta. The use of these agents increased the demands for iron, and there was renewed focus on iron management.

There are, however, specific aspects of anemia management that are more relevant to the elderly dialysis population. These include many other causes of anemia in the elderly population in general but still relevant for the dialysis patient. The prevalence of hematological conditions, particularly myelodysplastic syndrome, is much increased in the older patient, as are many cancers. Thus, anemia management in the elderly may be somewhat complex, and resistance to ESA and iron therapy is common. Poor diet and nutritional deficiencies are also more common in the elderly. The remainder of this chapter will discuss the prevalence and causes of anemia in the elderly, ESA therapy, iron management, and the role of blood transfusions. Specific attention will be given to the use of ESA therapy in patients with a previous or current history of stroke or malignancy, as well as a discussion on how to manage the patient who is resistant to ESA therapy.

Prevalence of Anemia in the Elderly

The incidence and prevalence of anemia increase with age. Using the World Health Organization definition of anemia (hemoglobin <13 g/dL for men and <12 g/dL for women), 11.0 % of men and 10.2 % of women aged 65 years or older and living in the community were anemic, according to the Third National Health and Nutrition Examination Study (NHANES III) data set [3]. The prevalence of anemia increases sharply in later life to values of 26.1 % in men and 20.1 % in women aged 85 years and over [3].

A high prevalence of anemia was also found in a longitudinal Swedish study of elderly subjects followed at 1–5 year intervals for 18 years [4], as well as a cross-sectional study of community-dwelling older persons in the Chianti area of Italy (CHIANTI Study) [5]. Much higher prevalences of anemia in the elderly dialysis population are seen, with upward of 95 % of patients being anemic or requiring treatment with ESA therapy.

The implications of anemia in the elderly population are severalfold. There are strong associations with a number of unfavorable outcomes that include death, functional dependence, dementia, falls, and cardiovascular disease. There are also economic implications for anemic individuals, with healthcare costs (both direct and indirect) being substantially higher in anemic patients compared to those without anemia.

Causes of Anemia in the Elderly

The major causes of anemia in the elderly, both in nondialysis and dialysis patients, are erythropoietin deficiency and iron deficiency (Table 9.1). Even without chronic kidney disease, elderly patients are known to have inappropriately low levels of erythropoietin for the degree of anemia, and it is estimated that approximately 30 % of anemia in the elderly is due to relative or absolute erythropoietin deficiency [6]. In approximately 50 % of cases, anemia in the elderly is due to reversible causes, including iron, B_{12}, and folate deficiency [6]. Chronic inflammation [6] and blood loss (which may be occult and secondary to malignancy) are also very common in the elderly and may also exacerbate anemia in this age group. There is a direct relationship between the prevalence of myelodysplastic syndrome and aging (clinical clues include a raised mean cell volume (MCV), resistant anemia, and abnormally low white cell and platelet counts). Hematinic deficiencies such as those associated with iron, B_{12}, and folate are easily diagnosed and treated, as is hypothyroidism which often presents with a macrocytic anemia. Gastrointestinal inflammation such as gastritis, esophagitis, and duodenitis, as well as peptic ulceration, may result in occult bleeding from the GI tract. Some drugs may also have anemia as a side effect and exacerbate this condition (Table 9.1).

Iron deficiency is also fairly common in the elderly and particularly so in dialysis patients. This may be due to a combination of both decreased iron intake and increased iron losses (Fig. 9.1), and thus, the dialysis population is often found to be in a state of negative iron balance. Iron absorption from the gut is severely impaired due to hepcidin overactivity as a result of increased inflammation [7], and certain commonly used drugs such as proton pump inhibitors and phosphate binders may bind to iron and impede iron absorption. Tea and certain foodstuffs may also have the same effect. In addition to iron losses caused by occult or overt GI bleeding, there may be iron losses due to blood trapping in the dialyzer, as well as secondary to frequent blood sampling. Use of aspirin as cardiovascular prophylaxis and heparin or other anticoagulants on hemodialysis may exacerbate gastrointestinal blood and iron losses.

Malignancy is much commoner in the elderly, and this may exacerbate anemia both by causing blood loss (e.g., bowel cancer) and by exacerbating chronic

Relative erythropoietin deficiency
Iron deficiency
B_{12} and/or folate deficiency
Chronic inflammation
Blood loss
Gastrointestinal inflammation (gastritis, esophagitis, duodenitis)
Malignancy
Myelodysplastic syndrome
Hypothyroidism
Drug side effects

Table 9.1 Causes of anemia in the elderly

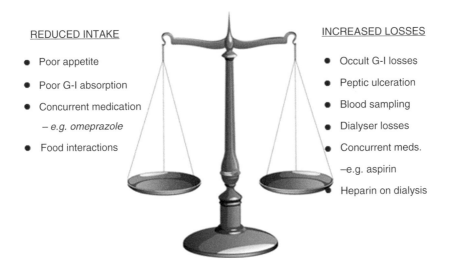

REDUCED INTAKE

- Poor appetite
- Poor G-I absorption
- Concurrent medication
  - *e.g. omeprazole*
- Food interactions

INCREASED LOSSES

- Occult G-I losses
- Peptic ulceration
- Blood sampling
- Dialyser losses
- Concurrent meds.
  - e.g. aspirin
  - Heparin on dialysis

Fig. 9.1 Iron balance in dialysis patients

inflammation (also known as the anemia of chronic disease) [6]. Caution is required in using ESA therapy in patients with current or previous malignancy (see below).

Erythropoiesis-Stimulating Agent (ESA) Therapy

The first-generation ESAs were epoetin alfa and epoetin beta, introduced in the early 1990s. Use of these agents revolutionized the management of anemia in dialysis patients, rendering many individuals free of blood transfusions and causing a sustained increase in the hemoglobin concentration [1, 2]. In hemodialysis patients, epoetin may be administered either intravenously or subcutaneously at a dosing frequency of one to three times per week. In peritoneal dialysis patients, the epoetin is virtually always given subcutaneously.

Subcutaneous administration of epoetin generally results in dose requirements that are 20–30 % lower than those seen with intravenous administration [8].

In 2001, a second-generation ESA was approved for the management of anemia in dialysis patients, called darbepoetin alfa (Aranesp®). The elimination half-life of darbepoetin alfa given intravenously is approximately three times that of epoetin (25.3 h vs 8.5 h). This agent is therefore able to be administered with less frequent injections, usually once per week or once every 2 weeks. In contrast to epoetin, there is no difference in dosing requirements between intravenous and subcutaneous administration with darbepoetin alfa.

A third-generation ESA has also been produced by inserting a polyethylene glycol (PEG) molecule into the epoetin molecule. Pegylated epoetin beta (methoxy polyethylene glycol epoetin beta or CERA; brand name Mircera®) has a much longer half-life than all the other ESAs, at around 130 h. This allows the agent to be injected once every 2 weeks, or even once a month. Again, there is no difference between intravenous and subcutaneous dosing requirements. For patent reasons, this product has not been able to be marketed in the United States, but it is widely available throughout Europe and the rest of the world. A randomized controlled trial (PATRONUS) showed superiority of pegylated epoetin beta compared to darbepoetin alfa when administered once–monthly to dialysis patients [9].

Most dialysis patients are already on ESA therapy by the time they start dialysis, but not infrequently there are "crash-landers" who present to their nephrologist with end-stage renal failure and often quite severe anemia which requires dialysis and ESA therapy.

Since ESAs were introduced, there has been much debate and controversy about the appropriate target hemoglobin range to aim for in dialysis patients. Following all the early studies which aimed for incomplete correction of anemia, interest then arose in completely normalizing the hemoglobin concentration. A large randomized controlled trial in hemodialysis patients comparing a target hemoglobin of around 14 g/dL with a hemoglobin of around 10 g/dL [10], however, was the first of several studies in the setting of chronic kidney disease to suggest that this strategy of anemia management may be harmful. There was an increased incidence of vascular access thrombosis in the group of patients targeting a normal hemoglobin concentration, and there was also a trend toward a higher risk of reaching the primary endpoint of death or a nonfatal myocardial infarction [9]. Several subsequent studies in nondialysis patients, including CREATE [11], CHOIR [12], and TREAT [13], have also raised concerns about normalization of hemoglobin. The latter study in particular has had the greatest impact on anemia management, and the latest anemia guidelines suggest that subnormal correction of anemia is preferable, with a target hemoglobin of around 10–12 g/dL. In the TREAT Study, aiming for a hemoglobin concentration of around 13 g/dL resulted in a doubling of stroke risk and a more than tenfold increase in cancer-related mortality in patients who had a previous malignancy [13]. Given that stroke and cancer are much more prevalent in the elderly population, this has significant implications for the use of ESA therapy in elderly dialysis patients (discussed in greater detail below).

ESA Therapy and Stroke

The incidence of stroke rises progressively with age, and thus, this devastating cardiovascular event is very much more common in the elderly patient. There are real concerns that ESA therapy may exacerbate the risk of stroke if a hemoglobin target of around 13 or 14 g/dL is implemented, and two randomized controlled trials have provided evidence to that effect.

The first trial was in hemodialysis patients recruited from across Europe and Canada [14]. Although the absolute number of strokes in the trial was low, there were nevertheless 12 strokes seen in the group of patients targeting a higher hemoglobin concentration of over 13 g/dL, compared to only four strokes in the group of patients targeting a hemoglobin concentration of around 10 g/dL ($p=0.045$) [14]. The TREAT Study of over 4000 patients with diabetes and nondialysis chronic kidney disease [13] showed a doubling of stroke risk in the group of patients targeting a hemoglobin of 13 g/dL, compared with the placebo group who maintained hemoglobin concentrations of just above 9 g/dL. Overall 154 of the 4038 patients included in this study had a stroke, with 101/2012 (5.0 %) in the active arm and 53/2026 (2.6 %) in the placebo arm (hazard ratio 1.9; 95 % confidence interval 1.4–2.7) [13].

The data from the TREAT Study were subjected to a further detailed analysis to see if any baseline variables could account for the development of stroke in the study population. A multivariate logistic regression model was used to identify baseline predictors of stroke. A number of other factors, including post-randomization blood pressure, hemoglobin level, platelet count, or treatment dose, were also assessed using a nested case-control analysis (1:10 matching) identifying non-stroke controls with propensity matching to see if any of these factors could account for the increased risk related to ESA therapy [15]. None of the baseline variables or any of the factors in the case-control analysis could be used to mitigate the risk of ESA-related stroke. Although the absolute risk of stroke was greater if there was a history of previous stroke, the relative risk of stroke in patients treated with ESA therapy remained at 2:1 versus placebo [15].

It is still not clear why ESA therapy might exacerbate stroke, but it is clear ESAs produce circulating erythropoietin levels that are considerably higher than physiological levels and that there are pleiotropic effects of these agents [16]. Thus, the increased risk of stroke may not be due simply to a higher hemoglobin concentration but to some of the secondary effects of ESA therapy, perhaps their effect on endothelial and platelet function.

The implications of all of this for anemia management are that physicians using ESA therapy should be aware of the potential for exacerbating stroke and in any patients believed to be high risk, the benefits versus the risks of using this treatment should be weighed up carefully. If ESA therapy is used, target hemoglobin concentrations should not exceed 11.5 or 12 g/dL in order to reduce the risk of this potentially devastating adverse effect.

ESA Therapy and Malignancy

Since the introduction of ESA therapy, there have been increasing concerns about the use of this treatment in patients with a history of previous or current cancer. The main concerns center around three main areas, namely, an increased risk of venous thromboembolism and whether there is any increased risk of death or tumor progression.

Most of the oncology trials using ESA therapy showed that targeting hemoglobin concentrations greater than 12 g/dL doubles the risk of venous thromboembolism. This complication is already increased in patients with cancer but appears to be further exacerbated by ESA therapy. In the CKD setting, in noncancer patients, the only trial that has been large enough to systematically look at the risk of this complication has been the TREAT Study, where again a doubling of the rate of venous thromboembolism was seen [13]. Again, this may be due to the pleiotropic effects of ESA therapy on endothelial and platelet function [16], but the consistency across all the oncology studies in various different types of cancer is harder to ignore.

The mortality risk in patients with malignancy is somewhat less clear. One of the earliest oncology trials of erythropoietin therapy for anemia associated with head and neck cancer suggested that patients whose tumor tissue tested positive for the erythropoietin receptor had a worse survival form those who were negative for the erythropoietin receptor [17]. This work has, however, since been discredited.

However, the publication of the TREAT Study once again raised concerns about the possibility of ESA therapy exacerbating cancer-related death. Patients with active malignancy were excluded from this study, although those who had a previous malignancy from at least 5 years ago and were deemed to be cured could be recruited. In this latter subgroup of patients, analysis of the rate of cancer-related death was conducted, and there was a more than tenfold increase in ESA-treated patients compared to the placebo group [13]. Given that this was not the primary objective of the study, the result needs to be interpreted with caution, although the magnitude of this effect is hard to ignore.

The question of whether ESA therapy can exacerbate the growth of a malignant cell clone is even more controversial. While the main function of erythropoietin is as a growth factor for red cells, there has been much discussion as to whether ESA therapy can also enhance tumor cell growth. This issue is still undecided.

All of the above has resulted in the physician not knowing what to do when a dialysis patient develops cancer. Given the uncertainty, it is perhaps sensible to use the lowest dose of ESA therapy possible, although these are the very patients who often show the greatest resistance to ESAs. Repeated dose escalation should therefore be avoided, and it may have to be accepted that patients on dialysis with an active cancer require red cell transfusional support. If ESA therapy is used, efforts should again be made not to target hemoglobin concentrations above 12 g/dL.

Hyporesponsiveness to ESA Therapy

There are two types of poor response to ESAs. The first is a failure to show a significant increment in hemoglobin concentration, despite repeated increases in ESA doses. The second is characterized by a loss of response to treatment, again despite increased ESA doses. The latter is more common in dialysis patients, although the former may occur in "crash-lander" patients who present with end-stage renal failure with no previous nephrological input. Hyporesponsiveness to ESA therapy should be subjected to a careful and systematic approach, and a cause for this should be rigorously sought. Common causes include iron insufficiency, infection or inflammation, and under-dialysis, while there are a number of less common causes

(Table 9.2). In the elderly dialysis patient, blood loss, B_{12} or folate deficiency, and a primary bone marrow disorder such as myelodysplastic syndrome may be more apparent than in a younger individual.

Investigating a patient who is hyporesponsive to ESA therapy merits a stepwise approach (Fig. 9.2). If the patient is self-injecting, then adherence with the prescribed treatment should be questioned and confirmed. The reticulocyte count may give a clue as to whether there is a primary problem with erythropoiesis, or whether the bone marrow is already working effectively, thus suggesting a shortened red cell survival as a result of bleeding or hemolysis.

The possibility of either absolute or functional iron deficiency (see below) should be considered, and if there is any doubt, then a trial of increased intravenous iron may be helpful. A raised C-reactive protein may suggest active infection or malignancy, particularly in the elderly, and this should be vigorously investigated. Occult

Table 9.2 Causes of a poor response to ESA therapy

Common	Less common
Iron deficiency	B_{12}/folate deficiency
Inflammation (infection/malignancy)	Hemolysis
Blood loss	Marrow disorders, *e.g., myelodysplastic syndrome*
	Under-dialysis
	ACE inhibitors
	Hypothyroidism
	Anti-EPO antibodies (PRCA)

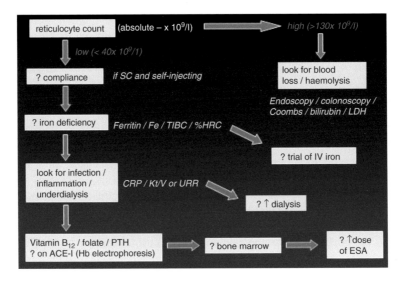

Fig. 9.2 Investigation of a poor response to ESAs

conditions such as tuberculosis or malignancy should also be considered, although these may prove somewhat elusive to detect. An increase in dialysis prescription and/or a change from conventional hemodialysis to hemodiafiltration may be of benefit. Screening for vitamin B_{12} or folate deficiency, blood loss, or hemolysis may be indicated, particularly in the elderly. A sharp fall in hemoglobin coupled with a very low reticulocyte count should alert the physician to the very rare condition of antibody-mediated pure red cell aplasia. Bone marrow examination may be required to exclude some hematological conditions such as myelodysplastic syndrome, very common in the elderly. A higher reticulocyte count makes it more likely that bleeding or hemolysis is the cause and a full hematinic screen and possible gastrointestinal investigations may be indicated (Fig. 9.2).

Whereas previously, physicians tended to escalate the dose of ESA therapy to higher and higher levels, recent randomized controlled trials have suggested possible harm in using high doses in ESA-resistant patients. It is still not clear whether the poor outcomes in this situation are due to the high doses of ESA therapy per se or whether this simply represents a group of patients who are generally more ill. Nevertheless, repeated dose escalation is no longer advised, and a maximum dose of epoetin of around 15,000 units per week in divided doses seems reasonable. This translates into a weekly dose of approximately 75 mcg of darbepoetin alfa or a monthly dose of approximately 300 mcg of pegylated epoetin beta.

Iron Management

Elderly patients are more prone to iron deficiency than their younger counterparts, and patients on dialysis are known to be in significant negative iron balance (Fig. 9.1). Thus, whereas healthy individuals lose 1–2 mg of iron per day via mucosal cell shedding in the gut, dialysis patients may lose up to four or five times this amount. Since dietary or orally administered iron is not absorbed due to hepcidin overactivity [7], intravenous iron has become mandatory in this patient population.

For the last two decades or so, iron deficiency has been categorized as being either *absolute* or *functional* (Table 9.3).

Absolute iron deficiency implies that there is a deficiency in total body iron stores, such that there are inadequate levels of iron to supply the bone marrow. The two types of iron deficiency are often compared to a bank account. Absolute iron

Table 9.3 Definition of absolute and functional iron deficiency

Absolute	Functional
Reduced body iron stores Low serum ferritin levels	Normal body iron stores but a failure to release iron rapidly enough to satisfy demands of bone marrow Normal/high serum ferritin ↓ Transferrin saturation (<20 %) ↑ Hypochromic red cells (>10 %)

deficiency implies that there is simply not enough money in the bank to be able to make a withdrawal.

Functional iron deficiency is a condition in which there are normal or even increased levels of total body iron stores, but there is a failure to mobilize this iron for use by the bone marrow for erythropoiesis. To continue the bank account analogy, functional iron deficiency is illustrated by a condition in which there is an ample amount of money in a savings account, but it cannot be withdrawn on demand.

Functional iron deficiency is much more common in the dialysis population, due to the chronic inflammatory state which upregulates hepcidin production by the liver (Fig. 9.3). Hepcidin is the master regulator of iron availability and its production is stimulated largely via interleukin-6 [7]. Hepcidin exerts its physiological effect by binding to the cellular iron export protein, ferroportin, thereby shutting down any iron efflux from cells responsible for iron transport, such as duodenal enterocytes, macrophages, Kupffer cells, and splenocytes [7]. The administration of intravenous iron circumvents the hepcidin-induced blockade of iron availability.

There are many laboratory tests available for the detection of iron deficiency, but none is ideal. The serum *ferritin* is a marker of body iron stores, and a very low serum ferritin level is diagnostic of absolute iron deficiency. Unfortunately, ferritin is also an acute phase protein and is elevated in chronic inflammatory states, as occurs almost ubiquitously in dialysis patients. Thus, a normal or even high ferritin level does not exclude the possibility of functional iron deficiency.

The *transferrin saturation* is also used as a marker of iron status, and levels of below 20 % are suggestive of iron insufficiency. However, levels of this parameter may fluctuate, and the absolute cutoff that will exclude functional iron deficiency or a response to additional intravenous iron is unclear.

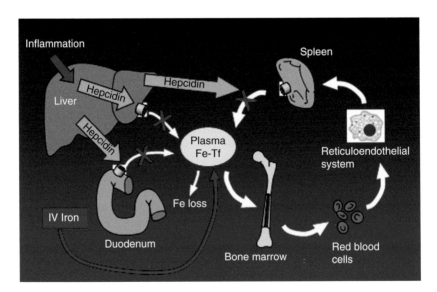

Fig. 9.3 Role of hepcidin in regulating iron supply in dialysis patients

The *percentage of hypochromic red cells* in the circulation has also been used as a marker of iron sufficiency but requires to be analyzed on a fresh sample. Thus, any delay in the sample reaching the laboratory may cause a serious elevation of this parameter. However, levels of <10 % should alert the physician to the possibility of iron insufficiency. Measurement of *reticulocyte hemoglobin content* uses a similar flow cytometric technique, with levels of <29 pg/cell suggestive of iron deficiency.

Since iron insufficiency is common in dialysis patients, supplementation of body iron stores is often required, and since this cannot be achieved by oral iron, intravenous iron replacement has become the standard of care in this population. Not only does this guarantee a readily available supply of iron, but it is extremely easy to administer to a hemodialysis patient who already has vascular access in situ. Thus, intravenous iron is usually administered during the dialysis session. There are many different intravenous iron preparations available worldwide. The older iron preparations such as iron dextran carry a small but definite risk of anaphylaxis due to preformed dextran antibodies; this has been found to be more prevalent with high-molecular-weight iron dextran compared to low-molecular-weight iron dextran compounds. Iron sucrose has been used for many years and has passed the test of time, being given to millions of patients worldwide. The usual administered dose is 100 or 200 mg, as tolerance at higher doses is reduced. Sodium ferric gluconate is also used in the dialysis population, mainly in the United States, Italy, and Germany. Several new intravenous iron preparations have recently been licensed, including ferric carboxymaltose, iron isomaltoside, and ferumoxytol. The main advantages of these preparations are that they can be administered in a higher dose over a shorter period of time, but their main applicability is in the nondialysis patient population. The amount of iron that dialysis patients require is not clear, but anemia guidelines suggest maintaining a serum ferritin level of somewhere between 200 and 500 ug/L, a minimum transferrin saturation of 20 %, and a minimum percentage of hypochromic red cells of 10 %. It is, however, clear that some patients respond to intravenous iron above these minimal thresholds, with an enhanced erythropoietic response. Whether or not this is harmful is not clear, and there are concerns that the liberal use of intravenous iron may exacerbate oxidative stress and infections. There is indeed evidence that intravenous iron administration may enhance bacterial proliferation and also reduce neutrophil function and for both of these reasons, IV iron should be withheld in patients with an acute bacterial or fungal infection.

Blood Transfusions

As outlined in the Introduction, blood transfusions were the mainstay of anemia management in dialysis patients prior to the introduction of recombinant human erythropoietin. Given the recent safety concerns with erythropoiesis-stimulating agents, however, there has been a recent increase in the use of transfusions in dialysis patients once again. In the elderly population, there is less concern about HLA sensitization than there is in the younger patient waiting for a kidney transplant, and there are also many conditions more prevalent in the elderly which can only be managed by intermittent transfusions (such as myelodysplastic syndrome and advanced hematological or solid-organ malignancy).

Blood transfusions also have a role in conditions causing sudden onset of anemia, such as acute blood loss or hemolysis. In patients who are septic and then become resistant to treatment with ESAs, blood transfusions may become necessary if the hemoglobin concentration becomes critically low.

There has been much debate over the years as to the trigger hemoglobin for administering blood during intercurrent illnesses, and the threshold has gradually decreased. Part of the reason for this is the outcome of several randomized controlled trials, which have not suggested any advantages in transfusing patients whose hemoglobin falls below 10 g/dL. There may even be harm in doing so, and the threshold for transfusion for stable conditions has fallen to around 7 g/dL. Indeed, a randomized controlled trial of two trigger hemoglobin concentrations for blood transfusion in the critical care setting (7 g/dL vs 10 g/dL) showed absolutely no benefit in transfusing patients at the higher hemoglobin trigger [18]. Even in the cardiac setting, when patients may be suffering from acute coronary syndrome, the use of blood transfusion above a hemoglobin level of 8 g/dL has been critically questioned. Thus, in the absence of acute bleeding, there is little indication to transfuse a patient above 7 or 8 g/dL unless a surgical procedure is planned in which significant blood loss might be expected.

Thus, in the modern era of anemia management, the focus is on the balance between ESA therapy, iron administration, and blood transfusions. The relative use of these three strategies should be selected for the individual patient, and many factors might influence this.

Conclusions

Anemia management in the elderly dialysis patient is not dissimilar to that in the younger subject and remains a balance among the use of ESA therapy, intravenous iron supplementation, and blood transfusions. There are, however, some specific differences that are relevant to the elderly population.

Nutritional deficiencies (vitamin B_{12}, folic acid, and particularly iron) are more common in the older patient, as is hypothyroidism. All of these deficiencies are easily corrected by the use of supplemental products. In the nondialysis setting, chronic inflammation is more common in the elderly, but whether this adds anything to the preponderance of inflammation induced by chronic dialysis is unclear. Blood loss may be more common in the elderly, as a result of gastrointestinal inflammation or malignancy. Several hematologic conditions are also more common in the elderly, and the most noteworthy of these is myelodysplastic syndrome which may be unresponsive to ESA therapy.

It is, however, likely that most patients will be treated with ESA therapy with or without supplemental intravenous iron and blood transfusions will be reserved for those resistant to these measures or when there is an intercurrent acute fall in the hemoglobin concentration.

The choice of hemoglobin target for the patient should also be individualized, in an attempt to maximize the benefits of anemia correction, while minimizing potential harmful effects. Thus, in patients with a previous stroke or malignancy, caution should be exercised in minimizing the use and dose of ESAs, given the concerns about possible exacerbation of these conditions with such agents.

Key Points
- Common causes of anemia in the elderly include erythropoietin deficiency, iron deficiency, B_{12} and/or folate deficiency, chronic inflammation, blood loss, gastrointestinal mucosal inflammation, malignancy, and myelodysplastic syndrome.
- A very low serum ferritin level (e.g., < 20 ug/L) conclusively proves a diagnosis of absolute iron deficiency – there is no other cause.
- The target hemoglobin concentration for elderly dialysis patients receiving ESA therapy should be individualized but should be somewhere around 10–12 g/dL.
- In patients showing a suboptimal response to ESA therapy, the reticulocyte count may provide helpful information. If low, then erythropoiesis is probably suppressed or deficient, whereas a high reticulocyte count might suggest bleeding or hemolysis.
- IV iron should not be given to patients with acute bacterial infection.

References

1. Winearls CG, Oliver DO, Pippard MJ, Reid C, Downing MR, Cotes PM (1986) Effect of human erythropoietin derived from recombinant DNA on the anaemia of patients maintained by chronic haemodialysis. Lancet 2:1175–1178
2. Eschbach JW, Egrie JC, Downing MR, Browne JK, Adamson JW (1987) Correction of the anemia of end-stage renal disease with recombinant human erythropoietin. Results of a combined phase I and II clinical trial. N Engl J Med 316:73–78
3. Guralnik JM, Eisenstaedt RS, Ferrucci L, Klein HG, Woodman RC (2004) Prevalence of anemia in persons 65 years and older in the United States: evidence for a high rate of unexplained anemia. Blood 104:2263–2268
4. Nilsson-Ehle H, Jagenburg R, Landahl S, Svanborg A (2000) Blood haemoglobin declines in the elderly: implications for reference intervals from age 70 to 88. Eur J Haematol 65:297–305
5. Cesari M, Penninx BW, Lauretani F, Russo CR, Carter C, Bandinelli S, Atkinson H, Onder G, Pahor M, Ferrucci L (2004) Hemoglobin levels and skeletal muscle: results from the InCHIANTI study. J Gerontol A Biol Sci Med Sci 59:249–254
6. Ferrucci L, Balducci L (2008) Anemia of aging: the role of chronic inflammation and cancer. Semin Hematol 45:242–249
7. Ganz T (2011) Hepcidin and iron regulation, 10 years later. Blood 117:4425–4433
8. Kaufman JS, Reda DJ, Fye CL, Goldfarb DS, Henderson WG, Kleinman JG, Vaamonde CA (1998) Subcutaneous compared with intravenous epoetin in patients receiving hemodialysis.

Department of Veterans Affairs Cooperative Study Group on Erythropoietin in Hemodialysis Patients. N Engl J Med 339:578–583

 9. Carrera F, Lok CE, de Francisco A, Locatelli F, Mann JF, Canaud B, Kerr PG, Macdougall IC, Besarab A, Villa G, Kazes I, Van Vlem B, Jolly S, Beyer U, Dougherty FC, PATRONUS Investigators (2010) Maintenance treatment of renal anaemia in haemodialysis patients with methoxy polyethylene glycol-epoetin beta versus darbepoetin alfa administered monthly: a randomized comparative trial. Nephrol Dial Transplant 25:4009–4017
10. Besarab A, Bolton WK, Browne JK, Egrie JC, Nissenson AR, Okamoto DM, Schwab SJ, Goodkin DA (1998) The effects of normal as compared with low hematocrit values in patients with cardiac disease who are receiving hemodialysis and epoetin. N Engl J Med 339: 584–590
11. Drüeke TB, Locatelli F, Clyne N, Eckardt KU, Macdougall IC, Tsakiris D, Burger HU, Scherhag A, CREATE Investigators (2006) Normalization of hemoglobin level in patients with chronic kidney disease and anemia. N Engl J Med 355:2071–2084
12. Singh AK, Szczech L, Tang KL, Barnhart H, Sapp S, Wolfson M, Reddan D, CHOIR Investigators (2006) Correction of anemia with epoetin alfa in chronic kidney disease. N Engl J Med 355:2085–2098
13. Pfeffer MA, Burdmann EA, Chen CY, Cooper ME, de Zeeuw D, Eckardt KU, Feyzi JM, Ivanovich P, Kewalramani R, Levey AS, Lewis EF, McGill JB, McMurray JJ, Parfrey P, Parving HH, Remuzzi G, Singh AK, Solomon SD, Toto R, TREAT Investigators (2009) A trial of darbepoetin alfa in type 2 diabetes and chronic kidney disease. N Engl J Med 361: 2019–2032
14. Foley RN, Parfrey PS, Morgan J, Barré PE, Campbell P, Cartier P, Coyle D, Fine A, Handa P, Kingma I, Lau CY, Levin A, Mendelssohn D, Muirhead N, Murphy B, Plante RK, Posen G, Wells GA (2000) Effect of hemoglobin levels in hemodialysis patients with asymptomatic cardiomyopathy. Kidney Int 58:1325–1335
15. Skali H, Parving HH, Parfrey PS, Burdmann EA, Lewis EF, Ivanovich P, Keithi-Reddy SR, McGill JB, McMurray JJ, Singh AK, Solomon SD, Uno H, Pfeffer MA, TREAT Investigators (2011) Stroke in patients with type 2 diabetes mellitus, chronic kidney disease, and anemia treated with Darbepoetin Alfa: the trial to reduce cardiovascular events with Aranesp therapy (TREAT) experience. Circulation 124:2903–2908
16. Vaziri ND, Zhou XJ (2009) Potential mechanisms of adverse outcomes in trials of anemia correction with erythropoietin in chronic kidney disease. Nephrol Dial Transplant 24:1082–1088
17. Henke M, Laszig R, Rübe C, Schäfer U, Haase KD, Schilcher B, Mose S, Beer KT, Burger U, Dougherty C, Frommhold H (2003) Erythropoietin to treat head and neck cancer patients with anaemia undergoing radiotherapy: randomised, double-blind, placebo-controlled trial. Lancet 362:1255–1260
18. Hébert PC, Wells G, Blajchman MA, Marshall J, Martin C, Pagliarello G, Tweeddale M, Schweitzer I, Yetisir E (1999) A multicenter, randomized, controlled clinical trial of transfusion requirements in critical care. Transfusion Requirements in Critical Care Investigators, Canadian Critical Care Trials Group. N Engl J Med 340:409–417

Chapter 10
Dialysis in the Older Adult: Management of CKD–MBD

Martin K. Kuhlmann

Introduction

CKD–MBD is strongly associated with mortality and morbidity in the general dialysis population. The spectrum of clinical long-term consequences of CKD–MBD includes abnormal mineral metabolism; vascular, valvular, and soft-tissue calcifications; uremic bone disease; bone pain; and, last but not least, bone fractures. A consensus statement on treatment targets and principles for CKD–MBD in CKD and dialysis patients has been issued recently in the form of guidelines by the KDIGO group [1]. However, these guidelines do not specifically address specific treatment modalities in the subpopulation of elderly dialysis patients.

It is recognized by nephrologists that in dialysis patients >75 years of age, the focus may shift from prolonging life toward improving or maintaining quality of life and reducing disease-associated burdens. There are very few data on biochemical or medical factors predicting outcome in this specific population of elderly dialysis patients. The few studies available indicate that comorbidity and age become major determinants of outcome, while traditional factors, such as dialysis dose (Kt/V), hemoglobin levels, or duration of dialysis levels, have little or no predictive value [2]. The fact that classical outcome parameters appear to be less important in this population raises the question whether management of CKD–MBD in older dialysis patients should differ from that in younger dialysis patients.

In this chapter, special aspects of CKD–MBD care in older dialysis patients will be discussed. It is evident that individual treatment decisions in elderly patients need to be made with respect to the expected survival time, which can be estimated from validated models (www.touchcalc.com) based on comorbidities and current medical status and independent of age [3].

M.K. Kuhlmann, MD
Division of Nephrology, Department of Internal Medicine, Vivantes Klinikum im
Friedrichshain, Landsberger Alle 49, Berlin 10249, Germany
e-mail: Martin.kuhlmann@vivantes.de

© Springer Science+Business Media New York 2016
M. Misra (ed.), *Dialysis in Older Adults: A Clinical Handbook*,
DOI 10.1007/978-1-4939-3320-4_10

Epidemiology of CKD–MBD in Elderly Dialysis Patients

In the general dialysis population, mineral and bone disease is highly prevalent and well established as risk factor for both mortality and morbidity. With increasing age, the impact of CKD–MBD on outcome may theoretically change, but currently available data are insufficient to draw firm conclusions. Two European groups have reported on the spectrum of CKD–MBD in elderly dialysis patients. In the French ESRD population, elderly hemodialysis patients >75 years of age ($n = 3403$) exhibited lower serum phosphate and PTH concentrations but slightly higher calcium levels compared to HD patients <75 years of age ($n = 5766$). At the same time, the use of calcium-based and non-calcium-based phosphate binders as well as use of cinacalcet were significantly lower in the elderly population. The authors conclude that it appears easier to control laboratory parameters of CKD–MBD in elderly HD patients [4].

Similar results were reported from a Hungarian ESRD population, where a greater proportion of patients over the age of 65 years met KDIGO CKD–MBD targets while receiving less CKD–MBD-specific medication than younger patients. An inverse correlation between age and PTH levels was reported, indicating that hyperparathyroidism appears better manageable with increasing age. However, despite the apparently better control of CKD–MBD, the prevalence of bone disease and especially soft-tissue calcifications was higher in the older dialysis patients who also displayed significantly higher serum calcium levels. This was putatively explained by a higher proportion of older patients receiving calcium-based phosphate binders [5].

Taken these data together, it appears that CKD–MBD may be easier to control in older dialysis patients, which may be due to reduced dietary protein and phosphorous intake. On the other hand, nonspecific clinical signs and symptoms of MBD as well as tissue calcifications may be more prevalent in older patients due to a longer course of dialysis and a higher and longer comorbidity burden.

CKD–MBD in Elderly Dialysis Patients: Focusing on Bone Strength

In the older dialysis population, fractures secondary to CKD–MBD become more relevant when compared to younger patients. Compared with the general population, the overall incidence of bone fractures is significantly higher in the dialysis population, with the risk of hip fractures exceeding that of the general population by a factor of 4–14 [6]. More recent data indicate that elderly white dialysis patients appear to be at the greatest risk for fractures [7]. While the most common type of fracture in dialysis patients is pelvis/hip fracture, followed by vertebral, lower leg, and shoulder/arm fractures, the relative incidence of vertebral fractures increases with age. Because fractures are associated with a substantially increased risk for death and hospitalization, adequate measures need to be undertaken to reduce the fracture incidence in elderly dialysis patients [8, 9].

Multiple factors contribute to the increased fracture risk in dialysis patients including a large comorbidity burden, decreased physical strength due to protein-energy wasting and frailty with an increased susceptibility to falls. In addition, poly-pharmacy including centrally acting drugs, such as narcotics and psychoactive medication, may increase the likelihood of falls and fractures. Fractures following an inadequate trauma are typically a consequence of impaired bone strength and stability. In healthy individuals, both bone strength and stability (or fragility) depend on a well-regulated balance between bone formation and bone resorption. In most dialysis patients with CKD–MBD, this balance is heavily deranged resulting in lower bone strength and increased bone fragility.

Pathophysiology of Reduced Bone Strength

ESRD-related uremic osteodystrophy encompasses a spectrum of conditions that are classified based on histomorphometric criteria as osteitis fibrosa (high-turnover disease), mixed uremic osteodystrophy, osteomalacia (low-turnover disease), and adynamic bone disease. Chronically elevated PTH levels cause high bone turnover favoring bone resorption via direct and indirect activation of osteoclasts and osteo-blasts leading to osteitis fibrosa and potentially marrow fibrosis. Uremic osteodys-trophy may present clinically with bone and muscle pain, weakness, postural instability, and fractures [1].

Osteoporosis in the absence of CKD is a condition characterized by bone loss leading to reduced bone strength and an increased risk of fractures. The hip, spine, and wrist are most commonly affected. By histomorphometric criteria, osteoporosis is characterized by microarchitectural disruption and reduced bone quality. In women an earlier first phase of accelerated predominantly trabecular bone loss occurs during the perimenopausal period and is followed by a second period of accelerated cortical as well as trabecular bone loss occurring after the age of 70 [10]. In both genders numerous risk factors for the development of osteoporosis have been identified in addition to age (Table 10.1). Secondary causes of osteoporosis can be identified in more than 60 % of affected male patients [11]. Although there are experimental data suggesting that uremic toxins may cause a form of "uremic osteoporosis," the role of CKD as an independent risk factor for the development of osteoporosis remains controversial [12].

Due to the different pathophysiologic pathways, osteoporosis and renal osteo-dystrophy will coexist in the majority of older dialysis patients, especially in females. In these cases, low BMD may be associated with an enormous range of functional abnormalities of bone remodeling. A bone biopsy study in 98 middle-aged male ($n=63$) and female ($n=35$) dialysis patients revealed signs of osteoporo-sis with preferentially low bone formation in 46 % of the population [13]. Interestingly, osteoporosis was present in both low-turnover and high-turnover

Table 10.1 Risk factors associated with the development of osteoporosis

Endocrine disorders	*Medications*
Menopause	Glucocorticoids
Hyperparathyroidism	ACTH
Hypopituitarism (e.g., Sheehan's syndrome)	Cyclosporin
Growth hormone deficiency	Anticonvulsants (e.g., phenytoin)
Marfan syndrome	Thyroxine
Hypercortisolism	GnRH analogs
Hyperthyroidism	Heparin
Hypogonadism	Chemotherapy
Comorbid conditions	*Hematologic disorders*
Diabetes mellitus	Lymphoma
Gastrointestinal malabsorption	Leukemia
Gastrectomy	Multiple myeloma
Short bowel syndrome	Chronic hemolytic anemia
Chronic biliary obstruction	Systemic mastocytosis
Chronic systemic inflammation	
Rheumatoid arthritis	
Connective tissue diseases	
Inflammatory bowel disease	
Liver cirrhosis	*Miscellaneous*
Homocystinuria	Alcoholism
Hypercalciuria	Smoking
Organ transplantation	Vitamin D deficiency
	Immobilization
	Anorexia nervosa

Modified from Kansal and Fried [11]

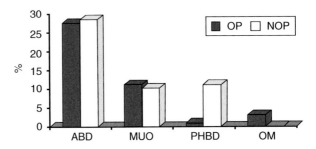

Fig. 10.1 Distribution of osteoporosis among ESRD-associated renal osteodystrophy. Results of a bone histomorphometry study in 98 maintenance hemodialysis patients [13]. *ABD* adynamic bone disease, *MUO* mixed uremic osteodystrophy, *PHBD* predominant hyperparathyroid bone disease, *OM* osteomalacia, *OP* osteoporosis, *NOP* non-osteoporosis

states, with the highest rate of osteoporosis occurring in patients with adynamic bone disease (Fig. 10.1). The relatively low rate of osteoporosis in predominantly hyperparathyroid bone disease patients may indicate that secondary hyperparathyroidism may to some degree be protective against trabecular bone loss. The real prevalence of osteoporosis in older dialysis patients is currently unknown, which is due to the methodological uncertainty in diagnosing osteoporosis in this population. However, it may be assumed that the prevalence of osteoporosis should be at least as high as in the general population of similar age but without kidney disease.

Diagnostic Evaluation of Bone Strength

Non-CKD Patients

In the general non-CKD population, there is a strong relationship between bone mineral density, bone strength, and fracture risk. Therefore, screening for osteoporosis is either based on measurement of bone mineral density (BMD) or on a history of osteoporotic bone fractures. There are various methods to assess BMD including central DEXA (dual-energy x-ray absorptiometry), peripheral DEXA (pDEXA), quantitative computer tomography, and quantitative ultrasound densitometry (heel ultrasound). Among these methods, central DEXA at the hip and spine is most frequently used to establish a diagnosis of osteoporosis and to predict future fracture risk. It is of note that DEXA can only assess overall density but not quality of the bone.

Independent of BMD, age, and other clinical risk factors, a radiographically confirmed vertebral fracture is a sign of impaired bone quality and strength and therefore consistent with the diagnosis of osteoporosis. Most vertebral fractures are asymptomatic when they first occur and often are undiagnosed for many years. Proactive vertebral imaging therefore is the only way to diagnose these fractures. Vertebral imaging is performed using a lateral thoracic and lumbar spine x-ray or by lateral vertebral fracture assessment (VFA), available on most modern DEXA machines at the time of BMD assessment. The presence of a single vertebral fracture is indicative for a fivefold increased risk for subsequent vertebral fractures and a two- to threefold risk of hip and any other fracture [14].

The value of serum biomarkers of bone remodeling for diagnosis of osteoporosis in the general population is not well established, but some of these may be useful for the assessment of individual responses to therapy. Biochemical markers of bone remodeling include resorption markers, such as serum C-telopeptide (CTX) and urinary N-telopeptide (NTX), and formation markers, such as serum bone-specific alkaline phosphatase, osteocalcin, and aminoterminal propeptide of type 1 procollagen.

The WHO definition of osteoporosis is based on bone mineral density (BMD) measurements, and most guidelines recommend screening DEXA in women >65 years and men >70 years or in postmenopausal women or men between 50 and 70 years with additional risk factors for fractures [15].

Elderly Dialysis Patients

Compared with the general population, assessment of bone strength in elderly dialysis patients is much more complex. In dialysis patients, the predictive value of BMD measurements is reduced due to the presence of renal osteodystrophy which renders the ability of BMD to predict fractures or other clinical outcomes in dialysis patients quite weak and inconsistent. Spine BMD may be overestimated by DEXA due to the presence of spinal osteophytes and aortic calcification in the area of measurement [16, 17]. In dialysis patients, BMD of the hip and radius is generally lower than in the general population, while lumbar spine BMD is similar to the non-CKD population. It must be recognized that forearm arteriovenous fistulae may negatively affect structure and growth of the nearby bone and, by decreasing values of BMD measurements, produce an overdiagnosis of osteoporosis [18]. If using peripheral DEXA in the radius region, the non-fistula arm should be studied. Although KDIGO guidelines do not recommend routine BMD testing in dialysis patients by any of the methods mentioned above, today, DEXA scan is most commonly used to assess BMD in dialysis patients. Besides that, the diagnosis of osteoporosis or low bone mass in dialysis patients is frequently made through demonstration of vertebral fractures by vertebral imaging or lateral abdominal radiographs.

Serum biomarkers of bone metabolism are affected by both renal osteodystrophy and osteoporosis and therefore are of little value for the diagnosis of osteoporosis in dialysis patients. Although high PTH levels may correlate with high-turnover bone disease, adynamic bone disease may prevail even in the presence of PTH levels between 100 and 500 pmol/l [1]. While there is an association of bone turnover markers and survival in the general dialysis population, the association of alkaline phosphatase with survival appears much weaker in older dialysis patients. In contrast, the association between PTH and mortality shows an opposite association. Thus, the effect of age needs to be considered when interpreting the prognostic implications of serum ALP and PTH levels [19].

Due to the reduced reliability of established diagnostic measures for BMD assessment in dialysis patients, iliac crest bone biopsy with double tetracycline labeling remains the gold standard for diagnosis of renal osteodystrophy and/or osteoporosis. Bone histology generates information about bone quality including turnover, mineralization, and volume. For a diagnosis of pure idiopathic osteoporosis, biopsy would be expected to reveal low trabecular bone volume and disrupted microarchitecture, without significant abnormalities in mineralization or bone turnover. In dialysis patients, these changes will be superimposed on CKD–MBD-specific alterations. Because of its invasiveness, bone biopsy is not a routine diagnostic step in the evaluation of CKD–MBD except in specialized centers. However, iliac crest bone biopsy should at least be considered in patients fulfilling one of the following criteria [20]:

- Occurrence of fractures with minimal or no trauma
- Intact PTH levels between 100 and 500 pmol/l with coexisting conditions such as unexplained hypercalcemia, severe bone pain, or unexplained increases in bone alkaline phosphatase
- Suspected aluminum bone disease
- Before the start of bisphosphonate therapy to exclude adynamic bone disease

Treatment of Dialysis Patients with Low Bone Mineral Density

The principal goal of CKD–MBD and osteoporosis therapy is improvement of bone mass and bone strength, which will translate in increased BMD. In idiopathic osteoporosis of the non-CKD patient, the pharmaceutical approach is primarily aimed at inhibiting osteoclastic bone resorption through bisphosphonates, estrogen, calcitonin, or raloxifene, mostly on top of standard calcium and vitamin D supplementation. With these antiresorptive strategies, a decrease in bone formation and an increase in bone mineralization can be observed which results in an increase in bone strength and BMD as well as in a reduction of low-trauma fracture rates by about 50 % [1]. The only anabolic substance currently used for osteoporosis treatment is recombinant human 1–34 PTH (teriparatide), which leads to an increase in BMD through induction of bone formation. A new therapeutic concept, which is currently undergoing clinical evaluation, is based on specifically inhibiting the action of sclerostin, an osteocyte-derived inhibitor of osteoblast activity through the monoclonal antibody romosozumab. Recently published results of a phase 2 trial showed an impressive increase in BMD and in bone formation [21].

The pathogenesis of bone disease in patients with CKD–MBD is different from that in postmenopausal osteoporosis; therefore, extrapolating results of studies from osteoporosis to dialysis patients may not be valid, especially with regard to long-term safety. Because until today no relevant clinical studies on treatment of low BMD in dialysis patients have been performed, treatment recommendations must be based on hypotheses and expert opinion. Similar to the non-CKD population, treatment principles in dialysis patients include non-pharmacologic and pharmacologic measures.

Non-pharmacological Treatment

Regular physical exercise remains the mainstay of any therapeutic or preventive approach to osteoporosis or low BMD. Especially in ESRD patients, who are exposed to prolonged phases of immobilization during dialysis treatment and in many cases throughout the whole treatment day, physical exercise is essential to stabilize or improve agility, strength, posture, and balance in order to prevent falls and subsequent fractures. Exercise may specifically suppress bone turnover and favor anabolic processes, even in adynamic bone disease. Regular weight-bearing and muscle-strengthening exercise should be recommended to reduce the risk of falls and fractures. Weight-bearing exercise (in which bones and muscles work against gravity as the feet and legs bear the body's weight) includes walking, jogging, Tai Chi, stair climbing, dancing, and tennis. Muscle-strengthening exercise includes weight training and other resistive exercises.

Excess alcohol consumption should be avoided. Alcohol intake of three or more drinks per day may be detrimental to bone health, increases the risk of falling and requires further evaluation for alcoholism when identified. Smoking cessation is also recommended.

Pharmacological Treatment

Calcium and Vitamin D

Calcium supplements and vitamin D are first-line therapies in non-CKD patients and may result in small increases in BMD but with uncertain effects on fracture rates [22]. In view of accelerated vascular and extravascular calcification processes in dialysis patients, daily calcium intake including the calcium load through calcium-based phosphate binders should not exceed an RDA of 1200 mg or even less in the presence of severe calcifications. 25-OH-vitamin D deficiency is common in elderly dialysis patients, related to impaired synthesis, inadequate intake, dietary restrictions, and low skin UV exposure. Dosage of active vitamin D should be carefully adjusted to avoid oversuppression of PTH and induction of adynamic bone disease.

Bisphosphonates

Bisphosphonates can be classified into two groups with different molecular modes of action: the simpler, nonnitrogen-containing substances clodronate and etidronate and the more potent nitrogen-containing compounds (alendronate, ibandronate, pamidronate, risedronate, and zoledronate). All bisphosphonates bind tightly to calcium in the hydroxyapatite crystal mineral with a half-life of up to 10 years. The major mode of action is related to inhibition of osteoclast activity or induction of osteoclast apoptosis, and it appears that in non-CKD patients, bisphosphonates are more effective in the presence of increased bone turnover [23].

In dialysis patients, where high bone turnover may be observed together with increased bone resorption, the use of bisphosphonates makes sense from a pathophysiological perspective. Indeed, in the few studies on the use of bisphosphonates in dialysis patients, it was shown that bisphosphonates may increase or stabilize bone density compared to placebo. In the largest randomized placebo-controlled trial in 31 hemodialysis patients, hip BMD remained stable after 6 months in alendronate-treated patients, compared with a reduction in placebo-treated controls. However, despite being significant, the difference was minimal, and treatment time was short [24]. Following bisphosphonate dosage, a transient increase in PTH levels has been described, which most likely is due to a short-term drop in serum calcium levels.

Bisphosphonates are recommended by some experts for dialysis patients with osteoporotic fracture types and a high risk for recurrent fracture [25]. However, it is uncertain whether low bone density alone, as in osteoporosis, is a sufficient indication for bisphosphonate therapy in dialysis patients. The risk in low-turnover osteopathy is that the bisphosphonate radically inhibits residual bone turnover, resulting in adynamic bone disease with an increased risk for fractures. Therefore, dialysis patients who might receive therapy would be those with low BMD but high bone turnover (osteitis fibrosa or mixed osteodystrophy). Since PTH levels alone do not allow differentiation of bone turnover rates [26], every dialysis patient would ideally need a bone biopsy before commencing bisphosphonate therapy.

The use of these bisphosphonates is formally contraindicated in patients with GFR < 30 ml/min and must be considered off-label use. Dosing of bisphosphonates therefore deserves special consideration in dialysis patients. While in non-CKD patients about half of the dose is eliminated via the kidney within several hours, virtually the entire bisphosphonate dose would be available to the bone in a dialysis patient. In dialysis patients, a dose reduction to 50 %, an extended dosing interval, and a maximum treatment period of 3 years are recommended.

Raloxifene

From a physiological point of view, the selective estrogen receptor modulator (SERM) raloxifene is expected to be beneficial to the bone in postmenopausal women with CKD–MBD. In non-CKD patients, it has been shown to reduce vertebral but not non-vertebral fractures [1]. The drug generally acts through estrogen receptors in the bone but is antagonistic to estrogen effects in the breast and uterus. A reduction in the risk of breast cancer therefore could be an additional benefit.

There are few studies on the use of this compound in female dialysis patients. One study demonstrates that after 1 year on raloxifene, postmenopausal women on hemodialysis had a significant increase in trabecular BMD and a decrease in bone resorption markers, suggesting that SERMs could constitute a therapeutic alternative to improve bone metabolism [27]. Because of an increased risk for deep venous thrombosis (DVT) and pulmonary embolism, SERMs should be avoided in women with a history of DVT. An increased risk of death from stroke was reported in postmenopausal women with coronary heart disease. Since the cardiovascular mortality risk in elderly women on dialysis is already increased, these agents should be used with caution in dialysis patients [1]. Further side effects are hot flashes and leg cramps.

Denosumab

Denosumab, a human monoclonal antibody directed against RANKL (receptor activator of NF-κB ligand), is a novel treatment for postmenopausal osteoporosis. Denosumab efficacy trials have not included dialysis patients. In the FREEDOM (Fracture Reduction Evaluation of Denosumab in Osteoporosis Every 6 Months) trial, a significant increase in BMD and a significantly lower risk of both vertebral and non-vertebral fractures was demonstrated in stage 3 CKD women treated with denosumab compared to placebo, and also the few subjects with stage 4 CKD appeared to accrue an increase in bone mineral density with denosumab [28].

Safety and efficacy of denosumab in end-stage renal disease is unclear. There is one case report of a female hemodialysis patient who developed severe hypocalcemia after a single subcutaneous injection of denosumab, which is biologically plausible because this agent neutralizes the RANKL receptor and thus reduces a signal that is essential for osteoclast formation, function, and survival. The decoupling of osteoclastic and osteoblastic activity may cause a net flux of calcium into the bone, especially in hyperparathyroid bone disease, where inhibition of osteo clast activity could result in a hungry bone-type syndrome [29].

Denosumab should be used with caution in hemodialysis patients due to the risk of severe hypocalcemia and lack of evidence supporting its efficacy in treating osteoporosis in this population. The fracture prevention efficacy of denosumab in dialysis patients still needs to be demonstrated.

Teriparatide

Studies in non-CKD patients have demonstrated the efficacy of recombinant human 1–34 parathyroid hormone (teriparatide) in the treatment of postmenopausal osteoporosis. However, patients with elevated baseline PTH levels were generally excluded from clinical trials. Thus, there are no data examining the efficacy of teriparatide in patients with evidence of hyperparathyroidism and CKD–MBD with potential peripheral PTH resistance. From a physiological perspective, the use of teriparatide might make sense in patients with adynamic bone disease and low PTH levels following parathyroidectomy [30]. But this concept needs further exploration in clinical studies. Use of teriparatide in elderly dialysis patients with low BMD cannot be recommended.

Calcitonin

Calcitonin has multiple physiological effects on the bone. It has been shown to inhibit osteoclast proliferation and decreases osteoclast activity, thereby inhibiting bone resorption increasing bone mineral content and improving bone architecture. Salmon calcitonin has been used to treat idiopathic osteoporosis. Due to a possible association between salmon calcitonin use and cancer incidence, it has been recommended recently to discontinue its use for treatment of osteoporosis [31].

Cinacalcet

The calcimimetic agent cinacalcet increases the sensitivity of the calcium-sensing receptor in the parathyroid gland to calcium, thereby downregulating parathyroid hormone levels. Use of cinacalcet may be associated with reduced bone turnover and improved bone histology. An almost 50 % reduction in bone fracture rates was reported from a combined analysis of the one phase 2 and three phase 3 randomized controlled clinical trials in 1184 patients with ESRD and uncontrolled hyperparathyroidism. Calcimimetics may act by ameliorating high bone turnover and increasing cortical bone mineral density and strength. These effects may be paralleled by favorable changes in biochemical markers of bone formation, such as BSAP, and bone resorption [32]. A decline in the incidence of hip fractures in HD patients aged older than 66 years has been observed during the period between 1993 and 2010, which coincided with an increased use of cinacalcet [33].

The recently published EVOLVE trial was designed to test the hypothesis that treatment with cinacalcet would reduce the risks of death and nonfatal cardiovascular events among patients with secondary hyperparathyroidism who were undergoing dialysis [34]. They did not show a significant advantage of cinacalcet in regard of the primary composite endpoint in the overall study population but did describe a significantly more pronounced effect of the drug among older patients. Data indicating a significantly lower fracture rate in cinacalcet-treated patients are contained in the supplementary appendix of the original publication. Further and more detailed evaluations are awaited. Taken these data together, it appears that favorable modulation of bone turnover by calcimimetics may result in a reduced fracture rate in dialysis patients.

Conclusion

The risk of fractures is significantly increased in dialysis patients and associated with increased risk of mortality and morbidity. Elderly dialysis patients should generally be viewed at high risk for reduced bone strength as a result of the combined effect of CKD–MBD and osteoporosis. Evaluation of bone strength is difficult in dialysis patients, especially because of a reduced predictive value of central or peripheral DEXA assessment. Vertebral radiography may be used to diagnose vertebral fractures as an indicator for reduced bone strength. Bone biopsy remains the gold standard to differentiate between osteoporosis and the various forms of renal osteodystrophy.

Preventive measures to increase bone strength include regular exercise and physical therapy to increase muscle mass and balance, maintaining a good nutritional status, and considerate pharmacological therapy including the use of calcimimetics, calcium, and vitamin D. Care needs to be taken to not oversuppress bone turnover, which may further increase bone fragility.

Basic therapeutic approaches in dialysis patients with low BMD and/or signs of osteoporosis include exercise and physical therapy as well as reduction of alcohol and nicotine consumption. Pharmacological options are few and mainly reserved for patients with low BMD and signs of high bone turnover. In these patients, moderate suppression of secondary hyperparathyroidism should be attempted by using vitamin D and/or calcimimetics. Low-dose and shorter-term bisphosphonates offer an alternative albeit off-label approach in these patients. Bone biopsy is recommended to exclude adynamic bone disease before prescribing bisphosphonates.

Key Points

1. In older female as well as male dialysis patients, age-related osteoporosis is frequently superimposed on the various forms of renal osteodystrophy resulting in loss of bone mass, reduced bone strength, and an increased risk of bone fractures.
2. The diagnostic value of biochemical markers for bone metabolism and of DEXA for assessment of bone mineral density is reduced, and the diagnosis of osteoporosis is frequently made through radiographic demonstration of vertebral fractures. Iliac crest bone biopsy remains the diagnostic gold standard technology.
3. Pharmacological treatment of CKD–MBD and osteoporosis should aim at inhibiting osteoclastic bone resorption while stimulating bone formation. Therefore, oversuppression of secondary hyperparathyroidism should be avoided.
4. Primary non-pharmacologic treatment measures include regular physical exercise, avoidance of excess alcohol consumption, and smoking cessation.
5. Patients with low bone mineral density and high bone turnover may benefit from the use of bisphosphonates and calcimimetics. Both substances may ameliorate high bone turnover and increase cortical bone mineral density and strength.

References

1. Kidney Disease Improving Global Outcome (KDIGO) CKD-MBD Work Group (2009) KDIGO clinical practice guideline for the diagnosis, evaluation, prevention, and treatment of chronic kidney disease – mineral and bone disorder (CKD-MBD). Kidney Int Suppl 76:S1–S130
2. Chauveau P, Combe C, Laville M et al (2001) Factors influencing survival in hemodialysis patients aged older than 75 years: 2.5 years outcome study. Am J Kidney Dis 37:997–1003
3. Cohen LM, Ruthazer R, Moss AH, Germain MJ (2010) Predicting six-month mortality for patients who are on maintenance hemodialysis. Clin J Am Soc Nephrol 5:72–79
4. Pelletier S, Roth H, Bouchet J-L et al (2010) Mineral and bone disease pattern in elderly hemodialysis patients. Nephrol Dial Transplant 25:3062–3070
5. Kiss I, Kiss Z, Ambrus C et al (2010) Age-dependent parathormone levels and different CKD-MBD treatment practices of dialysis patients in Hungary – results from a nationwide clinical audit. BMC Nephrol 14:155–162
6. Alem AM, Sherrard DJ, Gillen DL et al (2000) Increased risk of hip fractures among patients with end-stage renal disease. Kidney Int 58:396–399
7. Wagner J, Jhaveri KD, Rosen L et al (2014) Increased bone fractures among elderly United States hemodialysis patients. Nephrol Dial Transplant 29:146–151
8. Beaubrun AC, Kilpatrick RD, Freburger JK et al (2013) Temporal trends in fracture rates and post-discharge outcomes among hemodialysis patients. J Am Soc Nephrol 24:1461–1469
9. Tentori F, McCullough K, Kilpatrick RD et al (2014) High rates of death and hospitalization follow bone fracture among hemodialysis patients. Kidney Int 85:166–173
10. Berger C, Langsetmo L, Joseph L et al (2008) Change in bone mineral density as a function of age in women and men and association with the use of antiresorptive agents. CMAJ 178:1660–1668

11. Kansal S, Fried L (2010) Bone disease in elderly individuals with CKD. Adv Chronic Kidney Dis 17:e41–e51
12. Kazama JJ, Iwasaki Y, Fukagawa M (2013) Uremic osteoporosis. Kidney Int Suppl 3:446–450
13. Barreto FC, Barrto DV, Moyses RMA et al (2006) Osteoporosis in dialysis patients revisited by bone histomorphometry: a new insight into an old problem. Kidney Int 69:1852–1857
14. Lewiecki EM, Laster AJ (2006) Clinical applications of vertebral fracture assessment by dual-energy x-ray absorptiometry. J Clin Endo Metab 91:4215–4222
15. National Osteoporosis Foundation (2013) Clinician's guide to prevention and treatment of osteoporosis. National Osteoporosis Foundation, Washington, DC
16. Johnson DW, McIntyre HD, Brown A et al (1996) The role of DEXA bone densitometry in evaluating renal osteodystrophy in continuous ambulatory peritoneal dialysis patients. Periton Dial Int 16:34–40
17. Masud T, Langley S, Wiltshire P et al (1993) Effect of spinal osteophytosis on bone mineral density measurements in vertebral osteoporosis. BMJ 307:172–173
18. Muxí Á, Torregrosa J-V, Fuster D et al (2009) Arteriovenous fistula affects bone mineral density measurements in end-stage renal failure patients. Clin J Am Soc Nephrol 4:1494–1499
19. Letdumrongluk P, Lau WL, Park J et al (2013) Impact of age on survival predictability of bone turnover markers in hemodialysis patients. Nephrol Dial Transplant 28:2535–2545
20. Singh H (2009) Bone disease and calcium abnormalities in elderly patients with CKD. Am Soc Nephrol Online Curricula: Geriatric Nephrology, https://www.asn-online.org/education/distancelearning/curricula/geriatrics/Chapter14.pdf
21. McClung MR, Grauer A, Boonen S et al (2014) Romosozumab in postmenopausal women with low bone mineral density. New Engl J Med 370(5):412–420
22. Jackson RD, LaCroix AZ, Gass M et al (2006) Calcium plus vitamin D supplementation and risk of fractures. N Engl J Med 354:669–683
23. Toussaint ND, Elder G, Kerr PG (2009) Bisphosphonates in chronic kidney disease; balancing potential benefits and adverse effects on bone and soft tissue. Clin J Am Soc Nephrol 4:221–233
24. Wetmore JB, Benet LZ, Kleinstuck D, Frasetto L (2005) Effects of short-term alendronate on bone mineral density in hemodialysis patients. Nephrology (Carlton) 10:393–399
25. Miller PD (2007) Is there a role for bisphosphonates in chronic kidney disease? Semin Dial 20:186–190
26. Drueke TB (2008) Is parathyroid hormone measurement useful for the diagnosis of renal bone disease? Kidney Int 73:674–676
27. Hernández E, Valera R, Alonzo E et al (2003) Effects of raloxifene on bone metabolism and serum lipids in postmenopausal women on chronic hemodialysis. Kidney Int 63:2269–2274
28. Jamal SA, Ljunggren O, Stehman-Breen C et al (2011) Effects of denosumab on fracture and bone mineral density by level of kidney function. J Bone Miner Res 26:1829
29. McCormick BB, Davis J, Burns KD (2012) Severe hypocalcemia following denosumab injection in a hemodialysis patient. Am J Kidney Dis 60:626–628
30. Miller PD, Schwartz EN, Chen P et al (2007) Teriparatide in postmenopausal women with osteoporosis and mild or moderate renal impairment. Osteoporosis Int 18:59–68
31. Overman RA, Borse M, Gourlay ML (2013) Salmon calcitonin use and associated cancer risk. Ann Pharmacother 47:1675–1684
32. Cunningham J, Danese M, Olson K et al (2005) Effects of the calcimimetic cinacalcet HCl on cardiovascular disease, fracture, and health-related quality of life in secondary hyperparathyroidism. Kidney Int 68:1793–1800
33. Arneson TJ, Li S, Liu J et al (2013) Trends in hip fracture rates in US hemodialysis patients, 1993–2010. Am J Kidney Dis 62:747–754
34. The EVOLVE Trial Investigators (2012) Effect of cinacalcet on cardiovascular disease in patients undergoing dialysis. N Engl J Med 367:2482–2494

Chapter 11
Altered Pharmacology and Pill Burden in Older Adults: A Balancing Act

Darren W. Grabe and Katie E. Cardone

Introduction

Older adults represent one of the fasting growing age groups in many countries including the United States [1]. This rate of growth is mirrored in the dialysis population. The number of incident dialysis patients over the age of 65 years is greater than 50 %. The number of incident dialysis patients greater than 75 years of age represents the fasting growing population of dialysis patients.

This older dialysis population has consumed more medication over a similar time period. The increased medication use among older adults who are considered to be a vulnerable population demands scrutiny and careful attention [2–6]. This requires data-driven decision making to provide thoughtful medication management [7–9].

Unfortunately, most clinical studies do not include the elderly and exclude patients with CKD or receiving dialysis. As a result, there is a paucity of data to help guide clinical decision making in this vulnerable and complex population.

Altered Pharmacokinetics in Older Adults Receiving Dialysis

It is well recognized that older adults have physiologic changes as they age which influence the pharmacokinetics of drugs [10]. While the effect of some physiologic changes (decreased kidney function) is clear, other changes present more difficulty in establishing the clinical significance. Table 11.1 summarizes the perceived pharmacokinetic differences in older adults. Figure 11.1 represents a basic view of drug handling in the body along with the influence of kidney failure (Fig. 11.2).

D.W. Grabe, PharmD (✉) • K.E. Cardone, PharmD, BCACP
Department of Pharmacy Practice, Albany College of Pharmacy and Health Sciences,
Albany, NY, USA
e-mail: Darren.Grabe@acphs.edu

© Springer Science+Business Media New York 2016
M. Misra (ed.), *Dialysis in Older Adults: A Clinical Handbook*,
DOI 10.1007/978-1-4939-3320-4_11

Table 11.1 Pharmacokinetic differences in older adults

Variable	Change	Clinical implications
Absorption/ bioavailability	Reduced hydrochloric acid in stomach Reduction in gastrointestinal blood flow Decreased gastric motility and emptying Reduced lung alveolar surface area	Little
Volume of distribution	Increased for lipid-soluble drugs Decreased for water-soluble drugs Decreased lean body mass Lower albumin concentrations Reduced cardiac output	Increased half-life Higher plasma concentration Lower loading dose Increased free drug levels
Metabolism	Reduced hepatic blood flow Reduced number of hepatocytes	Increased half-life in phase I metabolism
Elimination	Decreased renal blood flow Decreased glomerular filtration rate	Increased half-life of renally excreted drugs

Fig. 11.1 Conceptual model of pharmacodynamics

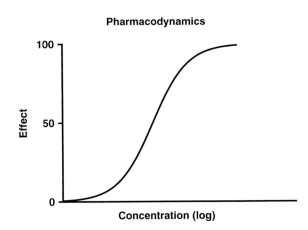

Absorption

Effect of aging: There are several age-related changes that may affect the absorption of drugs in older adults [11]. These include hypochlorhydria, altered splanchnic blood flow, and altered gastrointestinal motility. Hypochlorhydria is a natural process of aging and may result in a decreased dissolution of solid dosage forms of drugs administered orally. This, in turn, can lead to decreased absorption. First-pass metabolism decreases with age and may result in the increased absorption of drugs that are influenced by this process such as nitrates, beta blockers, and calcium channel blockers.

ESRD considerations: Absorption is affected in patients with ESRD due to changes in delays in gastric emptying, reduction in gastric acidity, interactions with phosphate binders, and changes in intestinal biotransformation and transport [12–14]. Delayed gastric emptying will modify the absorption profile of many orally administered medications and can result in lower peak concentrations and slower times to maximal absorption. Some medications require gastric acidity to

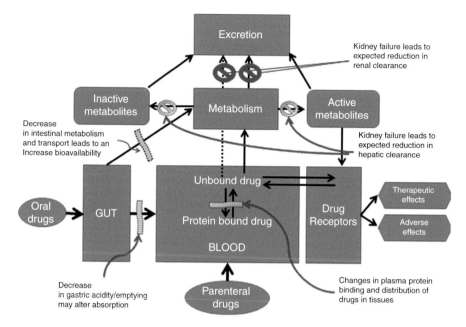

Fig. 11.2 Pharmacokinetic and pharmacodynamic alterations in older adults with kidney failure

maximize the dissolution of the dosage form, and thus, any reduction will likely have an impact on overall absorption of that medication, for example, oral iron preparations. Drug interactions with phosphate binders have been well established. This is particularly problematic for metal-based phosphate binders and coadministration with fluoroquinolones. Countering this is a decrease in intestinal metabolism and intestinal transport in patients with kidney failure. In kidney failure, changes at the cellular level affect drug absorption and subsequent bioavailability.

Clinical implications: The absorption profile of orally administered medications is affected by the aging process and kidney failure. Delays and reduction in overall bioavailability may be reduced, and patients may have a blunted response to certain medications.

Distribution

Effect of aging: A change in body composition occurs as individuals age. The most important change is an increase in body fat and a subsequent decline in both lean body mass and total body water [10]. In addition, many older adults may have a decrease in plasma protein binding.

ESRD considerations: The distribution of drugs is affected by kidney failure as a result of changes in volume status and decreased protein binding [15]. The overall changes in volume of distribution are complicated and difficult to predict. The volume of distribution of hydrophilic drugs may be increased in patients who have volume overload and decreased in those with muscle wasting. Plasma protein binding is reduced in patients receiving dialysis due to accumulation of uremic toxins, conformation changes in albumin, and hypoalbuminemia. The accumulation of uremic toxins has been shown to compete for binding sites on plasma proteins, thereby reducing overall protein binding of drugs. Changes in amino acid composition and carbamylation of albumin have been suggested and may contribute to decreased drug binding as a result of altered albumin composition. Hypoalbuminemia is a common finding in patients on dialysis and leads to a further reduction in plasma protein binding in these patients.

Clinical implications: Changes in drug disposition in older adults on dialysis will result in altered drug dosing. The volume of distribution of medications in older adults on dialysis will differ significantly from the general population. Increases in the unbound concentration of drugs coupled with a reduction in overall clearance will increase the likelihood of drug receptor binding.

Metabolism

Effect of aging: There is an age-related decline in overall liver volume as well as hepatic blood flow, and this has been implicated in reducing overall drug clearance [10, 16]. Hepatic blood flow may be decreased by as much as 40 % in older adults and, along with reduced blood volume, may predict reduced clearance of flow-dependent drugs or those with a high hepatic extraction ratio (e.g., morphine, propranolol, verapamil) [17]. Evidence supporting this claim is lacking with a high interindividual variability. Preliminary data in animal models show a decline in microsomal microenzymes; however, this has not been reliably duplicated in humans.

ESRD considerations: A decline in kidney function will result in a change in the hepatic clearance of drugs [14]. Inflammatory cytokines and certain uremic toxins such as parathyroid hormone and indoxyl sulfate are partially responsible for reducing cytochrome P450 (CYP) expression and enzymes (uridine diphosphate-glucuronosyltransferase and N-acetyltransferases) that mediate phase II reactions. Parathyroid hormone has been shown to reduce the expression of CYPs, specifically CYP3A, thereby reducing the hepatic metabolism of drugs that serve as substrates to that isoenzyme. Alterations in drug transport have been shown in experimental models of kidney failure with reductions in OATP expression of up to 40 % [15, 18]. A reduction in drug transport will lower overall metabolic clearance of drugs dependent on those pathways. Reduced renal metabolism of compounds should also be considered (e.g., vitamin D and insulin).

Clinical implications: Clinicians managing patients with kidney failure and receiving dialysis often focus on drugs that are renally cleared. Some attention to the impact of kidney disease and aging on hepatic function is warranted. Interventions such as control of secondary hyperparathyroidism and adequate dialysis have been shown to reverse some of the effects of kidney failure on hepatic drug clearance, but the results are unpredictable.

Excretion

Effect of aging: The potential for age-related declines in hepatobiliary clearance exists. Reductions in bile acid secretion and flow have been demonstrated and may impact the overall clearance of drugs and related metabolites [17].

ESRD considerations: The clearance on dialysis of drugs remains an important area of research as changes in dialysis modalities, technology, and new drugs enter clinical practice. Patients on intermittent hemodialysis exhibit two different elimination profiles: (1) intradialytic clearance, which occurs at a highly efficient rate during the dialysis session, and (2) interdialytic clearance, which represents the non-dialytic clearance achieved by both nonrenal mechanisms and any residual renal function. Thus, dosing of drugs should consider each of those scenarios. Increasing the time on dialysis or the number of sessions per week will impact overall drug clearance. A change in dialysis filter technology has also been shown to impact drug clearance with vancomycin as a prime example. Prior to the introduction of highly efficient, high-flux membranes, vancomycin was dosed once every 5–7 days. The more contemporary dosing of vancomycin represents the increased clearance achieved by modern membranes used in most dialysis centers.

Peritoneal dialysis is a modality that offers an attractive and viable option for older patients. The risk of hypotension is lower since it provides a more stable hemodynamic profile. It also minimizes transport issues of intermittent hemodialysis. Continuous ambulatory peritoneal dialysis (CAPD) provides continuous drug clearance but at a lower efficiency. Factors such as the dialysate flow rate (DFR) should be considered while prescribing and monitoring pharmacological therapy. Some medications may be administered intraperitoneally to reduce the need for another oral medication (e.g., antibiotics, vitamin D) or parenteral medications (e.g., antibiotics, insulin).

Clinical implications: Dialysis will have a significant impact on drug selection and dosing. Hemodialysis and peritoneal dialysis affect drug clearance in different ways. Clinicians should review available literature and existing guidelines on drug dosing in these settings. In the setting of dialysis, residual kidney function is often ignored, although the additional clearance thus provided may be significant. There are multiple drug information resources that provide guidance for choosing and selecting drugs in patients receiving dialysis.

Influence of Dialysis on Drug Dosing

Factors Affecting Drug Removal During Dialysis

Several factors may influence the clearance of drug molecules during dialysis. These include molecular weight, charge, protein binding, volume of distribution, water solubility, and the dialysis modality, filter characteristics, and dialysate and blood flow rates. In essence, drugs which have larger molecular weights, have significant protein binding, and have large volumes of distribution are less likely to be cleared efficiently during dialysis. The type of dialysis modality may also influence clearance (HD vs. PD). It is also important to note that the variants that exist within each of these modalities (e.g., CAPD vs. APD, traditional vs. extended hemodialysis treatments) will further affect the overall clearance of medications. However, studies outlining the specific pharmacokinetic profiles of individual agents in these settings and in older adults are limited. The advent of contemporary high-efficiency (large surface area) and high-flux (larger pore size) hemodialysis filters has increased the clearance of drugs. As such, drug dosing guidelines that reflect older technology (e.g., conventional filters) may provide inaccurate direction for optimal drug dosing.

Medications Commonly Administered at the Dialysis Facility

When evaluating a medication regimen for a patient on dialysis, it is important to note that a number of medications are commonly administered at the dialysis facility and are not self-managed. These medications may affect clinical outcomes, lead to drug interactions, and alter therapeutic decision making, yet may not be on a patient's home medication list. The typical medications that are administered at the dialysis facility include erythropoiesis-stimulating agents (ESAs), intravenous iron, vitamin D analogs, antimicrobials (vancomycin, cefazolin, ceftazidime, levofloxacin), and anticoagulants (heparin).

Altered Pharmacodynamics

Changes in Medication Responsiveness with Aging

The aging process will result in a change in receptor density, receptor affinity, signal transduction mechanisms, cellular response, and homeostatic regulation [19–22], ultimately leading to a diminished response to drugs that interact at those sites. The result is a change in the dose-response curve, making it more difficult to predict optimal dosing to achieve therapeutic targets while avoiding toxic doses. Thus, older patients respond differently to typical drug doses than younger patients. Age-related changes to body functions also contribute to variations in drug action. For example, blood supply to vital organs may be compromised through pathological processes (e.g., atherosclerotic narrowing of blood vessels). This may partially add to the increased sensitivity to centrally acting drugs such as benzodiazepines. Baroreceptor reflexes are decreased with age and can cause older adults to develop postural hypotension, making them prone to the adverse reactions of drugs that lower vascular smooth muscle action. Older adults will have lower plasma renin and aldosterone levels, which predisposes them to enhanced response to diuretics and calcium channel blockers and reduces response to beta blockers and drugs which act on the renin-angiotensin-aldosterone system (e.g., ACE inhibitors).

Pharmacodynamic Changes in the Cardiovascular System in Older Adults

Aging leads to a decreased response to adrenergic agents with a resultant decline in myocardial responsiveness to catecholamines and a decreased response to the chronotropic and inotropic effects of beta agonists [23]. Older adults require higher doses to elicit the same response seen in younger individuals with less tachycardia at similar doses. Conversely, older adults demonstrate greater sensitivity to beta blockers at similar doses. Plasma noradrenaline concentrations are increased with age and lead to downregulation of mediator responses. As an example, peripheral alpha blockers show similar pharmacokinetic profiles in younger and older adults, but elicit a greater reduction in blood pressure in older adults and a diminished relative rate of compensatory tachycardia [24].

Pharmacodynamic Changes in the Central Nervous System in Older Adults

In general, older adults are more sensitive to centrally acting pharmacological agents. Neurotransmission is markedly altered in older adults as a result of changes in structure, electrophysiological activity, and biochemical concentrations [25]. It is well known that aging decreases brain weight and gray matter volume, continuously accompanied by a loss of neuronal function [10]. Combined with a decrease in the number of synapses, changes in second messenger function (diacylglycerol, DAG) and neurotransmitter concentration (acetylcholine and dopamine) predispose older adults to adverse reactions to drugs that target those receptors.

Pharmacodynamic Changes in ESRD

Patients with ESRD are almost always excluded from dose-finding clinical studies that identify efficacious doses while minimizing adverse events. Because patients with ESRD are exposed to different ratios of parent drug and metabolites than patients with normal kidney function, it is unknown if the pharmacologic effect of the drug will differ compared with the general population. Additionally, the effect of uremia on medication use should be considered. For example, compromised immune function in patients with ESRD may require different antibiotic targets for efficacy (e.g., higher peak concentrations or more time over the minimum inhibitory concentration of the infecting organism). Because of impaired gluconeogenesis in ESRD, risk of hypoglycemia may be elevated with certain antidiabetic agents, even at doses adjusted for kidney function. Pharmacodynamic effects of medications in patients with ESRD are rarely well studied. Given the paucity of data in this area, caution should always be exercised when prescribing new medications to patients with ESRD.

Management of Common Diseases in Older Adults on Dialysis

Several special considerations are needed when managing conditions in older adults on dialysis. Changes in pharmacodynamic and pharmacokinetic drug profiles, along with multiple comorbidities and potentially frail individuals, create a challenging therapeutic landscape. Each section below outlines drug therapy considerations in this population.

Diabetes

There is a paucity of evidence to support treatment decisions in older adults with diabetes. In fact, a recent analysis has documented that most older adults have been excluded from clinical trials and that only 0.6 % of interventional trials targeted older adults ($\geq$65 years) [26]. The trials that did include older adults excluded patients on dialysis, resulting in a lack of clinical evidence to assist clinical decision making. Thus, the treatment of diabetes in older adults on dialysis is challenging and controversial, and clinicians caring for these patients must rely on extrapolating available evidence from clinical trials in different populations. It is also important to note that older adults often have various comorbid illness and disabilities that impact optimal diabetes control. For example, an older adult may suffer from functional disabilities such as vision loss, reduced manual dexterity, and/or cognitive impairment. Chronological age should not dictate therapy decisions, but should sensitize the clinician to consider alternate approaches to treatment and therapeutic goal setting. Optimal diabetes management must consider more flexible outcomes while avoiding significant hyper- and hypoglycemia. Hypoglycemia can result in devastating consequences in older adults. Older adults often have an altered response to hypoglycemia with impaired counter regulatory mechanisms leading to an elevated symptom threshold. Thus, regular blood glucose monitoring is critical. Since insulin is a commonly prescribed therapy for managing diabetes in patients on dialysis, clinicians should consider the hypoglycemia risk and adopt a pragmatic approach to dosing. Promoting the use of pen devices or insulin syringe magnifiers may help facilitate insulin administration. Clinicians may consider using intraperitoneal insulin for patients receiving peritoneal dialysis. There is one small study that expressed some concern of an increased risk of peritonitis with intraperitoneal insulin; however, the etiology of this remains undefined. Other concerns with intraperitoneal insulin administration that have been raised include dyslipidemia, subcapsular hepatic steatosis, and neoangiogenesis of the peritoneum [27–30]. Table 11.2 identifies preferred agents for managing diabetes in older adults on dialysis.

Table 11.2 Diabetes mellitus medications in aging patients on dialysis

Drug class	Use these…	Avoid these…	Notes
Alpha glucosidase inhibitors		• Acarbose[a] • Miglitol	• Lower efficacy than other therapies • Adverse GI reactions may limit use • Accumulation of parent molecules and their metabolites is a concern • These agents have not been studied in dialysis
Amylin analog		• Pramlintide	• Pramlintide significantly raises the risk of hypoglycemia and has not been studied in dialysis
Biguanide		• Metformin[a]	• Metformin is contraindicated in ESRD • Relative risk of lactic acidosis increased in patients over 80 years old
Dipeptidyl-peptidase-4 (DPP4) inhibitors	• Alogliptin • Linagliptin • Sitagliptin • Saxagliptin		• All require dosage adjustment in kidney failure except linagliptin with limited data in dialysis • Incidence of upper respiratory infections is 5 % This may potentially increase risk of other infections (e.g., peritonitis) in patients on dialysis • Linagliptin not excreted by dialysis and highly protein bound • Saxagliptin may worsen heart failure • Saxagliptin is removed by dialysis (23 %)
Incretin mimetics (GLP-1 agonists)	• Liraglutide • Albiglutide	• Exenatide	• No dosage adjustment necessary for liraglutide and albiglutide • Limited safety and efficacy data in kidney failure patients for liraglutide and albiglutide
Insulin, rapid acting	• Insulin lispro • Insulin aspart • Insulin glulisine • Insulin human powder (inhaled)		• Inhaled insulin I contraindicated in patients with asthma or COPD due to risk of acute bronchospasm

(continued)

Table 11.2 (continued)

Drug class	Use these…	Avoid these…	Notes
Insulin, short acting	• Insulin, regular		• May be added to peritoneal dialysis solution to manage diabetes • Avoid using sliding scale[b]
Insulin, intermediate acting		• Insulin, NPH	• Increased risk of hypoglycemia compared to long-acting insulins in older adults
Insulin, long acting	• Insulin detemir • Insulin glargine		• Basal insulins are preferred due to less chance of hypoglycemia in older adults
Meglitinides	• Repaglinide	• Nateglinide	• Initial dose of repaglinide should be reduced (0.5 mg with meals) • Nateglinide metabolites are active and may accumulate in kidney failure • Limited safety data exist for this class in kidney failure • Appear to be well tolerated in older adults
Others: bile acid sequestrant		• Colesevelam	• Colesevelam has a high pill burden and is structurally related to sevelamer, which the patient may already be taking Sevelamer also has the benefits of reducing lipids and A1C
Others: dopamine agonist		• Bromocriptine	• Not studied in patients on dialysis
Sodium-glucose cotransporter 2 (SGLT2) inhibitors		• Dapagliflozin • Canagliflozin • Empagliflozin	• SGLT2 inhibitors are likely not effective in patients with ESRD based on their mechanism of action
Sulfonylureas	• Glipizide • Glimepiride	• Glyburide[a,b] • Chlorpropamide[a,b] • Tolazamide[a] • Tolbutamide[a]	• Glyburide possesses a high risk of hypoglycemia in elderly and dialysis patients • 1st generation sulfonylureas are associated with cardiovascular risks
Thiazolidinediones	• Pioglitazone	• Rosiglitazone	• Rosiglitazone adversely affects lipids and is associated with poor cardiovascular outcomes • This class should be avoided in patients with heart failure

[a]Medication on PAIR Criteria List
[b]Medication on the Beer's Criteria List

Cardiovascular Conditions

Cardiovascular events remain the leading cause of death in patients on dialysis. This risk is significantly increased as patients age, with older adults over the age of 65 at the greatest risk. With respect to the management of heart failure or atrial fibrillation, the use of digoxin deserves special mention. Digoxin is primarily excreted by the kidney, and as such, the dosage should be appropriately adjusted to minimize the risk of toxicity. However, recent evidence suggests that the use of digoxin is associated with higher mortality rates in patients receiving hemodialysis [31]. This risk is dose related and further increased in the setting of low pre-dialysis serum potassium concentrations. Digoxin should be used with extreme caution in this population and only with strict monitoring of digoxin and potassium concentrations and patient symptomatology.

Hypertension

There are no uniform blood pressure therapeutic targets for patients on dialysis. The goal of treatment should be to minimize hypotensive episodes, while preventing spikes in blood pressure that could lead to stroke or other cardiac events. Blood pressure management should entail careful assessment of dry weight and fluid management in combination with medications. Both the choice of medications and the timing of medications should be considered when designing a regimen. If possible, at least one antihypertensive agent should be dosed at bedtime. With regard to the dialysis procedure, the dialytic removal of the drug should be considered as well as the pharmacodynamic effect of the drug during dialysis. Table 11.3 identifies preferred agents for managing hypertension in older adults on dialysis.

Dyslipidemia

Guidelines directed toward the general population promote the exclusive use of HMG-CoA reductase inhibitors for the management of dyslipidemia. However, current KDIGO guidelines do not support initiating treatment for dyslipidemia in patients on dialysis. However, if a patient was receiving drug therapy prior to dialysis, it may be continued. Dosage adjustment should be made based on kidney function. Drug interactions may be significant for this class. Simvastatin, lovastatin, and atorvastatin are metabolized by CYP3A4, and the use of strong inhibitors or inducers of CYP3A4 should be avoided concomitantly.

Thrombosis

The treatment of thrombotic conditions (e.g., atrial fibrillation) in older adults on dialysis presents some difficult challenges [32]. Despite the introduction of newer anticoagulants, warfarin and heparin serve as the mainstays for the management of these conditions. However, the use of warfarin in the dialysis population may be associated with increased risk for calciphylaxis and vascular calcification. Its use to treat atrial fibrillation is controversial in dialysis patients, given conflicting data.

Table 11.3 Antihypertensive medications in aging patients on dialysis

Drug class	Use these…	Avoid these…	Notes
Thiazide and thiazide-like diuretics	• Metolazone	• Hydrochlorothiazide • Chlorothiazide • Indapamide • Chlorthalidone	• Thiazides may be efficacious in patients with anuria, as they reduce peripheral vascular resistance • If used, metolazone is commonly prescribed in combination with loop diuretics to enhance diuresis
Loop diuretics[a]	• Furosemide • Torsemide • Bumetanide	• Ethacrynic acid	• Use only in non-anuric patients • Ethacrynic acid is more likely to cause ototoxicity than other loop diuretics • [a]Avoid use in older adults for dependent edema only
Aldosterone antagonists		• Spironolactone[b] • Eplerenone	• Preliminary data suggest the use of spironolactone may be beneficial in patients on dialysis; however, studies are ongoing
Beta blockers and alpha-beta blockers[a,c]	• Atenolol • Bisoprolol • Carvedilol • Labetolol • Metoprolol tartrate • Metoprolol succinate • Nebivolol	• Acebutolol • Betaxolol • Nadolol • Pindolol • Propranolol • Timolol	• Increased risk of bronchospasm in patients with COPD • Atenolol is removed by hemodialysis (50 %) but has favorable outcomes when dosed three times per week after hemodialysis • Preliminary data suggest that carvedilol has antioxidant properties and may confer cardioprotection in patients on dialysis • Nebivolol requires a reduction in dose for dialysis but has not been studied • Nebivolol has a lower incidence of sexual dysfunction • Nebivolol has a vasodilatory effect
Calcium channel blockers (non-DHP)	• Diltiazem[a,b] • Verapamil[a,b]		• [b]Non-DHP CCBs should be avoided in older adults with chronic constipation • Avoid combination with beta blockers • [a]Avoid use with NYHA class III or IV heart failure
Calcium channel blockers (DHP)	• Amlodipine • Felodipine • Isradipine • Nicardipine • Nifedipine (XL) • Nisoldipine	• Nifedipine (IR)	• May cause gingival hyperplasia which may affect denture fit in older adults • Immediate-release nifedipine is associated with profound hypotension precipitating myocardial infarction
ACE inhibitors	• Benazepril • Enalapril • Fosinopril • Lisinopril • Perindopril • Quinapril • Ramipril • Trandolapril	• Captopril	• Select medication based on intradialytic blood pressure (if hypertensive, use an ACE inhibitor that is not removed by dialysis – fosinopril or benazepril, if hypotensive select an agent that is removed by dialysis) • Captopril is dosed TID, which may lead to poor adherence • ACE inhibitors are removed by dialysis except for fosinopril and trandolapril

Table 11.3 (continued)

Drug class	Use these…	Avoid these…	Notes
ARBs	• Azilsartan • Candesartan • Eprosartan • Irbesartan • Losartan • Olmesartan • Telmisartan • Valsartan		• ARBs are not removed by dialysis
Direct vasodilators[a]	• Minoxidil • Hydralazine		• Hydralazine requires dosage adjustment in ESRD • Minoxidil use in women may lead to unwanted hypertrichosis • [a]*Increased risk of syncope and falls in older adults*
Direct renin inhibitor		• Aliskiren	• Very limited data on the use of aliskiren in ESRD
Alpha antagonist		• Doxazosin[b] • Prazosin[b] • Terazosin[b]	• Alpha blockers cause significant orthostasis in older adults and offer inferior cardiovascular protection compared with other classes
Central alpha agonists	• Clonidine[b]	• Reserpine • Methyldopa	• Avoid the use of this class in older adults when possible; increases risk of bradycardia and orthostasis

DHP dihydropyridine, *IR* immediate release, *ACE* angiotensin-converting enzyme, *ARB* angiotensin receptor blocker
[a]Medication on the STOPP Criteria List
[b]Medication on the Beer's Criteria List
[c]Medication on PAIR Criteria List

The direct thrombin inhibitor (i.e., dabigatran) is renally eliminated and may pose significant safety concerns in dialysis patients. There is also no reliable reversal strategy in the setting of severe bleeding. Factor Xa inhibitors (i.e., apixaban, rivaroxaban, and fondaparinux) have not been studied in patients on dialysis. Rivaroxaban and fondaparinux unnecessarily increase bleeding risk in patients with chronic kidney disease. The safety and efficacy have not been established for apixaban in older adults with ESRD. However, a reduced dosage may be considered. Nadroparin and tinzaparin are approved by the US Food and Drug Administration for use during hemodialysis to prevent clotting.

Pain Syndromes

Pain is a common clinical condition in patients on dialysis, which is often undertreated. In fact, the prevalence rate is approximately 50 %, with 74 % of those with moderate to severe pain not receiving any analgesia [33]. The management of pain in older adults on dialysis is particularly difficult since many agents adversely affect functional status. Pain medications may worsen cognitive function, increase fall risk and subsequently increase fall-related morbidity and mortality, negatively impact gastrointestinal integrity, and increase the risk of cardiovascular events. The World Health Organization's analgesic ladder has been proposed as a simplistic approach to pain relief. However, it ignores neuropathic pain and only offers oral medications for consideration. A modification of the WHO analgesic ladder has been proposed for patients with ESRD which eliminates NSAIDs and COX-2 inhibitors in step 1, codeine in step 2, and morphine in step 3. Consideration of topical agents should be incorporated in any management plan to avoid untoward, adverse effects of oral agents. Finally, non-pharmacological therapy may be useful for some patients, with high-tone external muscle stimulation a potential option for patients with neuropathic pain. Table 11.4 identifies preferred agents for managing pain in older adults on dialysis.

Neuropsychiatric Conditions

Older adults on dialysis are at risk for a multitude of neuropsychiatric conditions including depression, dementia (e.g., Alzheimer's disease), Parkinson's disease, sleep disturbances, and insomnia. These conditions are particularly difficult to

Table 11.4 Pain medications in aging patients on dialysis

Drug class	Use these…	Avoid these…	Notes
Opioid analgesics[a]	• Hydromorphone (IR) • Hydrocodone • Tramadol[b]	• Fentanyl • Meperidine[b,c] • Methadone • Morphine • Hydromorphone (ER) • Oxycodone • Pentazocine[b]	• Meperidine metabolite (normeperidine) accumulates in kidney failure and causes neurotoxicity • Methadone and meperidine associated with highest risk of falls in older adults • Methadone requires dosage adjustment in ESRD, not removed by HD • Fentanyl associated with most expensive injury-related ED visits in older adults • Morphine and oxycodone removed by dialysis • [b]Tramadol lowers the seizure threshold and concomitant use with SSRIs and TCAs should be avoided • Tramadol dosage adjustment necessary in older adults and dialysis • [a]*Avoid long-term use in older adults (risk of drowsiness, postural hypotension, vertigo)*

Table 11.4 (continued)

Drug class	Use these…	Avoid these…	Notes
NSAIDs[a,b,c], salicylates, and acetaminophen	• Acetaminophen • Diclofenac (topical) • Methyl salicylate (topical) • Trolamine (topical)	• Acetylsalicylic acid[a,b] • *Celecoxib*[a] • Choline magnesium salicylate[a] • Diclofenac[a, b] • Diflunisal[a,b] • Etodolac[a,b] • Fenoprofen[a, b] • Flurbiprofen[a,b] • Ibuprofen[a,b] • Indomethacin[a,b] • Ketoprofen[a,b] • Ketorolac[a,b] • Mefenamic acid[a,b] • Meclofenamate[a,b] • Meloxicam[a,b] • Nabumetone[a,b] • *Naproxen*[a,b] • Oxaprozin[a,b] • Piroxicam[a,b] • *Salsalate*[a] • Sulindac[a,b] • Tolmetin[b]	• NSAIDs should generally be avoided to protect residual kidney function and to avoid gastric irritation, bleeding, and ulcers. Celecoxib and salsalate may be associated with lower risk • NSAIDs are associated with increased cardiovascular risk. Indirect and observational data suggest that naproxen has a lower risk of adverse cardiovascular events compared to other NSAIDs • Use of NSAIDs should be limited to short term or with a proton pump inhibitor or misoprostol • [b]Aspirin >325 mg per day • *[a]Aspirin >150 mg per day* • *[a]NSAIDs to be avoided in older adults with history of* • Peptic ulcer disease • GI bleeding (w/o therapy) • Moderate-severe HTN • Heart failure
Adjunctive agents	• Gabapentin[c] • Nortriptyline • Pregabalin[c]	• Duloxetine • Amitriptyline[a,b] • Chlordiazepoxide • Clomipramine[a,b] • Doxepin[a,b] • Imipramine[a,b] • Perphenazine[a,b] • Trimipramine[a,b]	• [c]Gabapentin requires dosage adjustment in ESRD and is removed by dialysis • Duloxetine and metabolites accumulate in kidney failure • Tertiary TCAs are highly anticholinergic and sedating and cause orthostatic hypotension in the elderly • Nortriptyline may be inappropriate in those with a history of falls • [c]Pregabalin requires dosage adjustment in dialysis
Skeletal muscle relaxants		• Baclofen • Carisoprodol[b] • Chlorzoxazone[b] • Cyclobenzaprine[b] • Metaxalone[b] • Methocarbamol[b] • Orphenadrine[b]	• Skeletal muscle relaxants are highly anticholinergic and sedating, making them poor choices for elderly patients

NSAID nonsteroidal anti-inflammatory drug, *TCA* tricyclic antidepressant agent, *IR* immediate release, *ER* extended release
[a]Medication on the STOPP Criteria List
[b]Medication on the Beer's Criteria List
[c]Medication on PAIR Criteria List

manage in the non-dialysis patient and become more difficult in the setting of kidney failure. Among the selective serotonin reuptake inhibitors (SSRIs), fluoxetine and sertraline are preferred in patients on dialysis. As an added benefit, sertraline may be used for intradialytic hypotension. It should be noted that SSRIs can increase bleeding risk through their effects on platelet aggregation. Tricyclic antidepressants should be avoided due to cardiovascular risks and anticholinergic side effects. Benzodiazepines should be avoided whenever possible; however, lorazepam is preferred when one is necessary. For Alzheimer's disease, cholinesterase inhibitors may be used in dialysis with the exception of galantamine. Parkinson's disease medications may also be used to treat restless leg syndrome in patients on dialysis. Some examples include drugs like carbidopa/levodopa, pramipexole, and catechol-O-methyltransferase inhibitors.

Nutritional Supplements

Malnutrition that occurs in approximately 40 % of older adults on dialysis is a significant risk factor for mortality [34]. Various approaches to managing malnutrition have been investigated and include pharmacological interventions such as megestrol acetate and dronabinol and non-pharmacological interventions with protein bars, liquid-based supplements (e.g., Nepro), and intra-dialytic parenteral nutrition. Megestrol acetate is not recommended for use in this population based on inconsistent data supporting its effectiveness and significant adverse effects (adrenal insufficiency, venous thromboembolism) associated with its use.

Gastrointestinal Conditions

Many patients on dialysis have gastrointestinal conditions that require treatment. These management decisions in the setting of an older adult deserve additional considerations to avoid unwanted adverse effects. Fluid consumption should be considered when selecting medications for constipation. For example, caution should be exercised when using polyethylene glycol powder and bulk-forming laxatives. Electrolyte-containing laxatives such as sodium phosphate and magnesium citrate should be avoided. Medications to treat diarrhea with anticholinergic properties should be avoided, such as tincture of opium, paregoric, and diphenoxylate/atropine. Most antiemetics and antinausea agents are highly anticholinergic and should be avoided in older adults. Metoclopramide may be used for gastroparesis but can cause extrapyramidal side effects. Proton pump inhibitors are preferred for gastroesophageal reflux disease and ulcers, but may be associated with an increased risk for osteoporosis-related fractures of the hip, wrist, or spine. Sucralfate should be avoided in dialysis due to aluminum content.

Genitourinary Conditions

Older adults often develop genitourinary conditions including prostatism, benign prostatic hyperplasia, and urinary incontinence. However, as these patients initiate dialysis and urine production is reduced to an anuric level, it is important to recognize the opportunity to discontinue those related medications. This intervention has the benefit of reducing medication burden and minimizing cost and related adverse effects. This approach also holds true for diuretics, which lose effectiveness once the patient develops anuria.

Complications of ESRD

Anemia

Anemia is likely to be multifactorial in older adults on dialysis, requiring the clinician to consider vitamin deficiencies such as vitamin B12 and folate. Poor management of anemia in these patients will compromise functional status, contribute to cognitive impairment, and increase risk of falls and fall-related complications [35, 36]. Subcutaneous administration of ESAs may be more difficult given changes in subcutaneous fat disposition in older adults. As such, clinicians should monitor clinical response to these agents since pharmacokinetic profile may be altered.

Bone and Mineral Metabolism Disorders

Older adults on dialysis have multiple bone and mineral metabolism disorders that complicate typical management strategies. Osteoporosis is an important comorbidity in these patients, but its management is superseded by secondary hyperparathyroidism. It is also important to recognize that the use of bisphosphonates is contraindicated in patients on dialysis.

The use of phosphate binders is associated with poor compliance in the general dialysis population related to cost, pill burden, frequency of administration, and adverse effects [2]. These concerns are enhanced in older adults on dialysis. Clinicians must develop effective strategies to optimize therapy. Table 11.5 outlines some preferred agents for managing hyperphosphatemia in older adults on dialysis.

Table 11.5 Considerations in selecting a phosphate binder in aging patients on dialysis

Phosphate binder	Dosage forms	Advantages	Disadvantages
Sevelamer carbonate	• Tablet • Powder for suspension	• No exogenous calcium exposure • Reduces LDL cholesterol	• High pill burden • Expensive
Sevelamer HCl	• Tablet	• No exogenous calcium exposure • Reduces LDL cholesterol	• High pill burden • Expensive • Metabolic acidosis
Calcium acetate	• Capsule • Tablet • Solution	• Generic available • Multiple dosage forms	• Hypercalcemia
Lanthanum carbonate	• Chewable tablet	• Potent	• Expensive • Chewable tablet may be difficult for some older adults with poor dentition
Sucroferric oxyhydroxide	• Chewable tablet	• May reduce burden of parenteral iron • Potent	• Expensive • Chewable tablet may be difficult for some older adults with poor dentition
Calcium carbonate	• Various	• Inexpensive • Multiple dosage forms • Nonprescription	• Hypercalcemia
Aluminum hydroxide	• Suspension	• Potent • Inexpensive	• Chronic use associated with encephalopathy ("dialysis dementia") • Anemia • Bone disease
Tetraferric tricitrate decahydrate	• Tablet	• Potent, may reduce burden of parenteral iron	• Expensive, pill burden

Special Considerations Affecting Medication Use

Hemodialysis

Medication-related decisions should always consider the impact that hemodialysis has on therapy. A patient's hemodialysis schedule may dictate when certain medications can be administered. For example, some medications may be removed by dialysis, and thus, dosing may be reserved for after the session, while other drugs may be administered during dialysis to reduce overall pill burden when the patient is at home. Other changes induced by hemodialysis such as hypotension or cognitive changes may influence a patient's ability to take certain medications.

Peritoneal Dialysis

Peritoneal dialysis provides less efficient but continuous solute clearance. Clinicians should be cognizant of the type of dialysis and apply drug dosing recommendations appropriately. It is important to point out that there is limited evidence supporting dosing of drugs in peritoneal dialysis. Most available literature is related to antibiotics in continuous ambulatory peritoneal dialysis, with sparse data in more contemporary variants of peritoneal dialysis such as automated peritoneal dialysis. Finally, clinicians may consider intraperitoneal administration of drugs in dialysate; however, confirmation of stability and pharmacokinetic parameters should be studied prior to prescribing any such regimen.

Drug Prescribing in Older Adults

The elderly consume a disproportionately large number of drugs for multiple acute and chronic diseases. In fact, prescription medication consumption has increased substantially for numerous drug classes over the last two decades. Complicating the increase in prescription burden is a parallel increase in nonprescription drugs, with adults over 65 years old consuming 40 % of all nonprescription drugs [5]. Almost 90 % of older adults use nonprescription drugs, and this population uses twice as many nonprescription drugs as prescription drugs [5]. Accompanying the increase in medication burden are increases in costs to the patient and healthcare system. Average prescription drug costs for older Americans increased rapidly for many years, with average cost per person in the United States at $2834 in 2008. However, it is important to recognize that costs vary significantly among individuals. A small percentage (6 %) of older adults in the United States incurred no prescription drug costs in 2008, while more (15 %) incurred over $5000 in these costs. This variability can be partially explained by the presence of chronic conditions. For example, in 2008, an older adult with 5 or more chronic conditions paid over $5000 for prescription drugs compared to about $1200 in those with no chronic conditions. The increased use of medications is also associated with an increase in the risk of drug-related morbidity and mortality. Given the high number of comorbid conditions and associated prescription medications used in patients on dialysis, it is expected that they will fall in the highest cost category.

Polypharmacy and Inappropriate Medications

The issue of inappropriate medications in older adults has been addressed by using specific criteria to identify potentially inappropriate medications in older adults. The Beers' criteria are the most widely cited tool for this purpose. It was originally developed in 1991 and recently updated in 2012 [37]. The STOPP (Screening Tool of Older Persons' potentially inappropriate Prescriptions) criteria and START (Screening Tool to Alert doctors to the Right Treatment) criteria exist as two other tools to assist with evidence-based clinical decision making [38, 39]. Unfortunately, these tools are lacking in guidance for the management of older patients on dialysis. To address this deficiency, the PAIR (Pharmacotherapy Assessment in Chronic Renal Disease) criteria were developed in 2011 [40]. Utilizing each of these tools in concert may ultimately provide some insight into proper medication management in this vulnerable population.

Medication-Related Problems

Medication-related problems (MRPs) are common among patients who take ≥5 medications, take ≥12 medication doses per day, frequently change medications, have multiple disease states, are nonadherent, or use medications requiring therapeutic monitoring. Many patients with CKD meet all of these criteria, especially as CKD progresses to stage 5. For example, the average patient on hemodialysis requires 10–12 medications and has 6 comorbid conditions. Frequent review of the medication regimen is warranted in order to identify and resolve MRPs as well as keep an accurate medication list at all times. Inaccurate medication lists put patients at risk for MRPs. Analysis of one HD clinic electronic drug record demonstrated that 60 % of records contained at least 1 discrepancy [41]. These inaccuracies increased the risk of adverse drug events and dosing errors. In another similar study at an HD clinic, a 79 % discrepancy rate of reviewed records was reported. Reconciling medication lists is important for all patients, including those with CKD, as improving accuracy of the medication records allows proper intervention on MRPs.

Medication Regimen Complexity

Pill Burden

In a recent analysis the median daily pill burden in patients on dialysis was 19 with 25 % of the population taking greater than 25 pills per day [2]. Phosphate binders constituted nearly 50 % of this burden. This increased burden was associated with a decreased quality of life independent of the Charlson's comorbidity index. Medication regimen complexity is also a consideration in the care of patients with CKD and may impact adherence.

Medication Regimen Complexity Index

While some advocate for quantifying medication regimen complexity by counting the number of medications or the pill burden, these measures fall short of fully realizing the impact of other important variables such as multiple dosage forms, administration instructions, frequency, and specific restrictions related to specific medications. The Medication Regimen Complexity Index (MRCI) is a tool that has been validated in patients with respiratory disease, but has also been studied in dialysis patients [42]. Considering the full impact of the prescribed treatment regimen in a patient on dialysis must consider many factors including the quantity of medications, dosage forms, costs, frequency, timing, and collective adverse events.

Compliance/Adherence

There are significant barriers to successful adherence to medication regimens in older adults on dialysis [43]. As mentioned, patients on dialysis have complex medication regimens that carry a large pill burden along with special instructions. Administration of oral medications is difficult given the sheer number of pills but is complicated in these patients by the fluid restriction guidelines. Certain demographic and socioeconomic factors are also important variables to consider as many patients may have poorer adherence rates due to the cost of medications. Poor health literacy, chronic illness, cognitive impairment, and age may also contribute to limited recall or understanding of the prescribed regimens [44]. Older adults on dialysis may have poor vision and manual dexterity necessary for administering medications successfully.

Tips for Improving Medication Management

Disease state management should incorporate some basic approaches to maximize medication management and minimize barriers such as nonadherence, drug interactions, increased cost, and adverse drug reactions. These include taking a thorough medical, social, medication (including prescriptions, nonprescription drugs, and herbal supplements) history; consideration of the physiological effects of aging; conservative dosing and titrating to clinical therapeutic targets; communication with other healthcare team members; simplification of drug regimens to reduce complexity; introducing medication aids such as pill organizers to manage daily consumption; considering practical implications of drug storage containers and measurement of liquid volumes; and referring to appropriate drug information resources for possible drug and disease interactions [8, 9, 45].

Key Points/Summary
1. Pharmacokinetic changes commonly occur in both elderly patients and those with kidney impairment.
2. The combined influences of age, end-stage renal disease, and dialysis on medications are complex and may lead to unpredictable effects.
3. Patient characteristics such as age, life expectancy, patient priorities, quality of life, cognitive ability, health literacy level, and social circumstances should be taken into account when designing drug therapy regimens for elderly patients on dialysis.

References

1. Department of Health & Human Services AoA. U.S. Population by Age: July 1, 2010; 2010 [updated July 1 2010; cited 2014 1 Jul]
2. Chiu YW, Teitelbaum I, Misra M, de Leon EM, Adzize T, Mehrotra R (2009) Pill burden, adherence, hyperphosphatemia, and quality of life in maintenance dialysis patients. Clin J Am Soc Nephrol CJASN 4(6):1089–1096
3. Lassiter J, Bennett WM, Olyaei AJ (2013) Drug dosing in elderly patients with chronic kidney disease. Clin Geriatr Med 29(3):657–705
4. Olyaei AJ, Bennett WM (2009) Drug dosing in the elderly patients with chronic kidney disease. Clin Geriatr Med 25(3):459–527
5. Rolita L, Freedman M (2008) Over-the-counter medication use in older adults. J Gerontol Nurs 34(4):8–17
6. Larsen PD, Martin JL (1999) Polypharmacy and elderly patients. AORN J 69(3):619–622, 25, 27–28
7. Hubbard RE, O'Mahony MS, Woodhouse KW (2013) Medication prescribing in frail older people. Eur J Clin Pharmacol 69(3):319–326
8. Rifkin DE, Laws MB, Rao M, Balakrishnan VS, Sarnak MJ, Wilson IB (2010) Medication adherence behavior and priorities among older adults with CKD: a semistructured interview study. Am J Kidney Dis Off J National Kidney Found 56(3):439–446
9. Pai AB, Cardone KE, Manley HJ, St Peter WL, Shaffer R, Somers M et al (2013) Medication reconciliation and therapy management in dialysis-dependent patients: need for a systematic approach. Clin J Am Soc Nephrol CJASN 8(11):1988–1999
10. Hammerlein A, Derendorf H, Lowenthal DT (1998) Pharmacokinetic and pharmacodynamic changes in the elderly. Clinical implications. Clin Pharmacokinet 35(1):49–64
11. Bender AD (1968) Effect of age on intestinal absorption: implications for drug absorption in the elderly. J Am Geriatr Soc 16(12):1331–1339
12. Van Vlem B, Schoonjans R, Vanholder R, De Vos M, Vandamme W, Van Laecke S et al (2000) Delayed gastric emptying in dyspeptic chronic hemodialysis patients. Am J Kidney Dis Off J National Kidney Found 36(5):962–968
13. Van V, Schoonjans RS, Struijk DG, Verbanck JJ, Vanholder RC, Van B et al (2002) Influence of dialysate on gastric emptying time in peritoneal dialysis patients. Perit Dial Int J Int Soc Perit Dial 22(1):32–38
14. Joy MS, Frye RF, Nolin TD, Roberts BV, La MK, Wang J et al (2014) In vivo alterations in drug metabolism and transport pathways in patients with chronic kidney diseases. Pharmacotherapy 34(2):114–122
15. Naud J, Nolin TD, Leblond FA, Pichette V (2012) Current understanding of drug disposition in kidney disease. J Clin Pharmacol 52(1 Suppl):10s–22s

16. Schmucker DL (2005) Age-related changes in liver structure and function: Implications for disease? Exp Gerontol 40(8–9):650–659
17. Schmucker DL (1985) Aging and drug disposition: an update. Pharmacol Rev 37(2):133–148
18. Nolin TD, Frye RF, Le P, Sadr H, Naud J, Leblond FA et al (2009) ESRD impairs nonrenal clearance of fexofenadine but not midazolam. J Am Soc Nephrol JASN 20(10):2269–2276
19. Fleg JL, Schulman S, O'Connor F, Becker LC, Gerstenblith G, Clulow JF et al (1994) Effects of acute beta-adrenergic receptor blockade on age-associated changes in cardiovascular performance during dynamic exercise. Circulation 90(5):2333–2341
20. Fleg JL, Strait J (2012) Age-associated changes in cardiovascular structure and function: a fertile milieu for future disease. Heart Fail Rev 17(4–5):545–554
21. White M, Roden R, Minobe W, Khan MF, Larrabee P, Wollmering M et al (1994) Age-related changes in beta-adrenergic neuroeffector systems in the human heart. Circulation 90(3):1225–1238
22. Newgard CB, Pessin JE (2014) Recent progress in metabolic signaling pathways regulating aging and life span. J Gerontol A Biol Sci Med Sci 69(Suppl 1):S21–S27
23. Bowie MW, Slattum PW (2007) Pharmacodynamics in older adults: a review. Am J Geriatr Pharmacother 5(3):263–303
24. Andros E, Detmar-Hanna D, Suteparuk S, Gal J, Gerber JG (1996) The effect of aging on the pharmacokinetics and pharmacodynamics of prazosin. Eur J Clin Pharmacol 50(1–2):41–46
25. Peters R (2006) Ageing and the brain. Postgrad Med J 82(964):84–88
26. Dardano A, Penno G, Del Prato S, Miccoli R (2014) Optimal therapy of type 2 diabetes: a controversial challenge. Aging 6(3):187–206
27. Diaz-Buxo JA (2000) Use of intraperitoneal insulin with CCPD. Semin Dial 13(3):207
28. Nevalainen PI, Lahtela JT, Mustonen J, Taskinen MR, Pasternack A (1999) The effect of insulin delivery route on lipoproteins in type I diabetic patients on CAPD. Perit Dial Int J Int Soc Perit Dial 19(2):148–153
29. Quellhorst E (2002) Insulin therapy during peritoneal dialysis: pros and cons of various forms of administration. J Am Soc Nephrol JASN 13(Suppl 1):S92–S96
30. Torun D, Oguzkurt L, Sezer S, Zumrutdal A, Singan M, Adam FU et al (2005) Hepatic subcapsular steatosis as a complication associated with intraperitoneal insulin treatment in diabetic peritoneal dialysis patients. Perit Dial Int J Int Soc Perit Dial 25(6):596–600
31. Chan KE, Lazarus JM, Hakim RM (2010) Digoxin associates with mortality in ESRD. J Am Soc Nephrol JASN 21(9):1550–1559
32. Dager WE, Kiser TH (2010) Systemic anticoagulation considerations in chronic kidney disease. Adv Chronic Kidney Dis 17(5):420–427
33. Santoro D, Satta E, Messina S, Costantino G, Savica V, Bellinghieri G (2013) Pain in end-stage renal disease: a frequent and neglected clinical problem. Clin Nephrol 79(Suppl 1):S2–S11
34. Pasticci F, Fantuzzi AL, Pegoraro M, McCann M, Bedogni G (2012) Nutritional management of stage 5 chronic kidney disease. J Ren Care 38(1):50–58
35. Andres E, Serraj K, Federici L, Vogel T, Kaltenbach G (2013) Anemia in elderly patients: new insight into an old disorder. Geriatr Gerontol Int 13(3):519–527
36. Andro M, Le Squere P, Estivin S, Gentric A (2013) Anaemia and cognitive performances in the elderly: a systematic review. Eur J Neurol Off J Eur Fed Neurol Soc 20(9):1234–1240
37. American Geriatrics Society Beers Criteria Update Expert Panel (2012) American Geriatrics Society updated Beers Criteria for potentially inappropriate medication use in older adults. J Am Geriatr Soc 60(4):616–631
38. Gallagher P, O'Mahony D (2008) STOPP (Screening Tool of Older Persons' potentially inappropriate Prescriptions): application to acutely ill elderly patients and comparison with Beers' criteria. Age Ageing 37(6):673–679
39. Hamilton H, Gallagher P, Ryan C, Byrne S, O'Mahony D (2011) Potentially inappropriate medications defined by STOPP criteria and the risk of adverse drug events in older hospitalized patients. Arch Intern Med 171(11):1013–1019
40. Desrochers JF, Lemieux JP, Morin-Belanger C, Paradis FS, Lord A, Bell R et al (2011) Development and validation of the PAIR (Pharmacotherapy Assessment in Chronic Renal

Disease) criteria to assess medication safety and use issues in patients with CKD. Am J Kidney Dis Off J National Kidney Found 58(4):527–535

41. Manley HJ, Drayer DK, McClaran M, Bender W, Muther RS (2003) Drug record discrepancies in an outpatient electronic medical record: frequency, type, and potential impact on patient care at a hemodialysis center. Pharmacotherapy 23(2):231–239

42. George J, Phun YT, Bailey MJ, Kong DC, Stewart K (2004) Development and validation of the medication regimen complexity index. Ann Pharmacother 38(9):1369–1376

43. Browne T, Merighi JR (2010) Barriers to adult hemodialysis patients' self-management of oral medications. Am J Kidney Dis Off J National Kidney Found 56(3):547–557

44. Lee DS, de Rekeneire N, Hanlon JT, Gill TM, Bauer DC, Meibohm B et al (2012) Cognitive impairment and medication complexity in community-living older adults: the health, aging and body composition study. J Pharm Technol JPT Off Publ Assoc Pharm Tech 28(4):156–162

45. Power A, Brown E (2013) Optimising treatment of end-stage renal disease in the elderly. Nephron Clin Pract 124(3–4):202–208

Chapter 12
Dialysing the Elderly Patient with Congestive Heart Failure: What Is Important to Know?

Andrew Davenport

Introduction

The number of elderly patients surviving with increasing and more complex co-morbidity, especially in affluent countries, continues to grow exponentially. Elderly patients with the combination of chronic kidney disease stage 5 and congestive heart failure (CHF) have an increased risk of death. They should, if possible, be empowered to choose between conservative supportive care and dialysis. In countries without well-developed supportive palliative care programs, greater numbers of elderly patients with high co-morbidity scores, including CHF, withdraw from dialysis within the first few months of starting treatment [1]. This is particularly true for haemodialysis (HD). It is worth noting that a 4 h HD session may well expand into 8–10 h day, with the patient feeling too exhausted to do anything but to simply go to straight to bed on final arrival at home [2].

CHF

Many of the signs and symptoms of CHF result from sodium and water retention, i.e., leg swelling, orthopnoea, paroxysmal nocturnal dyspnoea, accompanied by the clinical signs of peripheral oedema, raised jugular venous pulse and pulmonary rales. However, these may simply represent an overhydrated dialysis patient. The echocardiogram and electrocardiogram (ECG) are the most useful tests to determine underlying cardiac pathology. The echocardiogram provides information on chamber volumes, left and right ventricular systolic and diastolic function, wall thickness and

A. Davenport, MD
UCL Center for Nephrology, University College London Medical School,
Royal Free Hospital, Rowland Hill Street, London NW3 2PF, UK
e-mail: andrewdavenport@nhs.net

© Springer Science+Business Media New York 2016
M. Misra (ed.), *Dialysis in Older Adults: A Clinical Handbook*,
DOI 10.1007/978-1-4939-3320-4_12

valve function, whereas the ECG primarily provides information regarding electrical conduction, chamber hypertrophy and loss of viable myocardium (Q waves). Measurement of natriuretic peptides has become standard practice in the general medical assessment of patients with suspected heart failure, with an N-terminal probrain natriuretic peptide (NTproBNP) concentration ≥300 pg/ml or brain natriuretic peptide (BNP) of ≥100 pg/ml (in the acute setting) and NTproBNP of ≥125 pg/ml or BNP of ≥35 pg/ml (in the chronic setting) suggestive of CHF. However, natriuretic peptide concentrations are normally higher in the elderly and may also be increased with chronic kidney disease, atrial arrhythmias, left ventricular hypertrophy and chronic obstructive pulmonary disease, thus making interpretation of single values less clear.

The majority of elderly dialysis patients will have some degree of ischaemic atheromatous cardiac disease (Table 12.1), due to the common underlying patho-

Table 12.1 Causes of heart failure in the elderly dialysis patient

Cardiac pathology	Causes
Coronary artery disease	Atheroma
	Arteriosclerosis
	Vasculitis
	IgG4 associated
Valvular heart disease	Degenerative
	Calcific
	Valve prolapse/dilatation valve ring
	Rheumatic fever
	Autoimmune diseases/vasculitis
	Syphilis
	Congenital
Myocarditis	Viral
	Endocrine (thyrotoxicosis)
Infiltrative	Sarcoidosis
	Malignancy
Hypertrophic cardiomyopathy	Hypertrophic obstructive cardiomyopathy
	Hypertension
	Amyloid
Dilated cardiomyopathy	Myocarditis
	Eosinophilic syndromes
	Iron overload
	Persistent overhydration
	High output arteriovenous fistula
Restrictive cardiomyopathy	Pericarditis (tuberculous)
	Amyloid
	Chemotherapy (anthracyclines)
	Endomyocardial fibrosis
	Anderson–Fabry
	Long vintage haemodialysis
Right ventricular heart failure	Secondary pulmonary hypertension
	High-output arteriovenous fistula
	Primary pulmonary hypertension

physiological mechanisms linking small vessel ischaemia and hypertension to the progression of chronic kidney disease. Nearly all elderly dialysis patients will have diastolic dysfunction (Table 12.2, adapted from ref [3]) that predisposes them to episodes of acute symptomatic heart failure typically precipitated by modest over-hydration or arrhythmias.

Haemodialysis is an independent risk factor for developing both de novo and recurrent heart failure, with 51 % mortality within 2 years after a diagnosis of CHF [4]. Besides heart failure, sudden arrhythmic death also accounts for a significant percentage of cardiac mortality in dialysis patients, and this appears to be tempo-rarily associated with the longer 72 h gap between dialysis sessions in the standard thrice-weekly schedule and is thought to be triggered by a combination of underly-ing abnormal ventricular morphology and function, electrolyte imbalances and overhydration [5].

Table 12.2 Echocardiographic assessment of systolic and diastolic myocardial function

	Abnormal parameter	Clinical relevance
Systolic dysfunction		
LV EF	<50 %	LV global dysfunction
LV fractional shortening	<25%	LV radial dysfunction
LV regional function	Akinesia, hypokinesia, dyskinesia	MI, ischaemia cardiomyopathy, myocarditis
LV end-diastolic size	Diameter ≥ 60 mm or >32 mm/m^2 or volume >97 mL/m^2	Volume overloaded
LV end-systolic size	Diameter >45 mm or >25 mm/m^2, or volume >43 mL/m^2	Volume overloaded
LV outflow tract velocity time integral	<15 cm	Reduced LV stroke volume
Diastolic dysfunction		
LV diastolic dysfunction	E/e ratio >15 E/A ratio >2	Severity and filling pressure
L atrial volume index	>34 mL/m^2	Increased LV filling pressure or mitral valve disease
LV mass index	Women >95 g/m^2 Men >115 g/m^2	Hypertensive heart disease, aortic stenosis, HOCM
RV		
TAPSE	<16 mm	RV systolic dysfunction
Systolic PAP	>50 mmHg	Pulmonary hypertension likely
IVC width	Dilated, no respiratory collapse	Volume overloaded, increased right atrial pressure, RV dysfunction

Adapted from European Society of Cardiology [3]
LV left ventricle, *RV* right ventricle, *EF* ejection fraction, *MI* myocardial infarction, *HF* heart fail-ure, *HOCM* hypertrophic obstructive cardiomyopathy, *TAPSE* tricuspid annular plane systolic excursion, *PAP* pulmonary artery pressure, *IVC* inferior vena cava

General Considerations for the Elderly Patient
with Congestive Heart Failure

Although there have been many randomised prospective drug trials in the field of CHF, typically both the elderly and patients with advanced chronic kidney disease have been excluded, and as such it is unclear whether the recommendations from these studies can be extrapolated to elderly dialysis patients. The pivotal trials which showed an advantage for beta-blocker therapy were conducted in patients with continuing symptoms of heart failure and a persistently low left ventricular ejection fraction, despite treatment with angiotensin-converting enzyme inhibitors (ACEIs) and, in most cases, combined with diuretics [6, 7]. The current cardiology consensus is that these treatments are complementary and that a beta-blocker and an ACE inhibitor, (or angiotensin receptor blocker if ACEIs cannot be tolerated) should both be started in low doses and titrated upwards according to clinical response and blood pressure [3]. ACE inhibitors generally only have a modest effect on LV remodelling, whereas beta-blockers often lead to a substantial improvement in ejection fraction and additionally are anti-ischaemic, reducing the risk of sudden cardiac death. Studies in haemodialysis patients with heart failure have reported a survival advantage with beta-blockers. However it is important that dialysis patients have their dry weight or target weight regularly reviewed and adjusted to minimise volume overload, as persistent hypervolaemia will exacerbate underlying cardiac dysfunction. Mineralocorticoid receptor blockers are recommended for patients with ongoing symptoms of heart failure but risk hyperkalaemia. However, several studies have reported that low doses of spironolactone can be given safely to chronic dialysis patients, if appropriately monitored [8].

It should always be recognised that excessive blood flow through an arteriovenous fistula or graft may exacerbate heart failure, and as such colour Doppler studies should be performed to regularly assess fistula flows, particularly with the increasing use of brachial fistulae and banding or other flow-restrictive procedures considered when flows are greater than 1.5 l/min.

If patients continue to suffer symptomatically with heart failure despite pharmacological therapy, and if the left ventricular ejection fraction is <35 % with a prolonged QRS complex, then resynchronisation pacemaker insertion may be helpful. However this should be discussed with a cardiologist as there is a significantly increased risk of bacterial colonisation and infection of the pacing leads in haemodialysis patients dialysing with a venous catheter and also in those using the button hole or constant site cannulation method for arteriovenous fistulae [9].

Supraventricular arrhythmias, particularly atrial fibrillation, are common in the elderly dialysis patient with CHF. Although digoxin is renally excreted, most patients can tolerate low doses without significant toxicity. The main debate in this area centres on the risk of stroke compared to bleeding between coumarin anticoagulants and aspirin [10]. Aspirin does increase the risk of gastrointestinal haemorrhage in the older patient, and it may be prudent to co-prescribe H2 blockers (as there is a potential increased risk of *Clostridium difficile* with proton pump inhibitors). Certainly in the non-dialysis population, warfarin therapy is more effective in reducing the risk of ischaemic stroke than aspirin. However the dialysis literature is less clear, with some studies reporting equal stroke prevention with both warfarin and aspirin, while others reporting reduced incidence of stroke but greater spontaneous bleeding with warfarin therapy. As such most clinicians continue to favour aspirin [11], although patient risks should be calculated on an individual basis to determine the likely risk–benefit of oral anticoagulation using scoring systems like CHA2DS2-VASc and HAS-BLED [12, 13].

Dialysis Choice for the Elderly Patient with Congestive Heart Failure

The options available for the older patient with CHF differ between health-care systems and from country to country. In the patients who have no available help, haemodialysis typically becomes the default option. Whereas if peritoneal dialysis can be performed by family members, or if the patient can receive assistance from visiting nursing staff or trained nursing home personnel, then peritoneal dialysis may well be the better option in terms of quality of life by reducing hospital or dialysis centre visits. Not surprisingly self-reported depression levels are high in elderly patients with chronic diseases. As such peritoneal dialysis patients without social support may become depressed and wish to withdraw from treatment, whereas in centre haemodialysis patients who have the opportunity to go outside their homes and meet other patients in the dialysis unit may be less depressed despite similar co-morbidity.

How Much Dialysis Does the Elderly Patient with CHF Need?

Clinical guideline committees have suggested minimum urea clearance targets for both haemodialysis and peritoneal dialysis patients. However these targets are based on historic cohorts of relatively younger and healthier patients studied in clinical trials. Body composition changes with age, so the older person has less skeletal muscle than when middle aged. Patients generally adapt their dietary intake according to physical activity, and it is recognised that patient activity declines with increasing co-morbidity. As such on one hand older dialysis patients with CHF would be expected to have a reduced dietary protein intake and do little if any exercise, thus reducing muscle (nitrogen) turnover and generating less nitrogenous waste products. On the other hand, CHF is an inflammatory state leading to cachexia. Thus it would appear that lower urea-based clearance targets might suffice, as many conservatively managed chronic kidney disease stage 5 patients remain relatively healthy until very shortly before their death. Indeed reducing the urea clearance target may well reduce disequilibrium symptoms in the older person and paradoxically improve patient wellbeing post-dialysis. Further studies are required to investigate energy expenditure and dialysis clearance targets for this group. The main indication for dialysis in these patients continues to be correction of overhydration.

Does the Elderly Patient with Congestive Heart Failure Need Dietary Supplements?

Water-soluble vitamins and other nutrients are lost during haemodialysis and hae-modiafiltration. Although there may be a marked fall in free serum levels during the dialysis session, there is no clinically significant clearance of water-soluble vitamins by different dialysis modalities, provided patients have an adequate diet [14]. However elderly dialysis patients with heart failure are unlikely to have adequate nutrition and would benefit from vitamin supplementation (water as well as fat soluble) [15]. Others have speculated about the need for carnitine supplementation, trace metals including zinc and selenium and other micronutrients in heart failure [16].

Peritoneal Dialysis for the Elderly Patient with Congestive Heart Failure

Peritoneal transport is traditionally described by the 3 pore model. Fast transporter status can either be due to increased peritoneal mesenteric capillary surface area or increased number of blood vessels. Patients with heart failure typically have an inflammatory milieu, due to oedema of the intestine, changes in gut permeability and increased endotoxin transfer [17]. As such most peritoneal dialysis patients with CHF behave as rapid transporters and may have difficulty achieving adequate ultrafiltration to correct their expanded extracellular volume, especially in an acute setting. Several studies which have reported clinical benefits and longer survival of patients with CHF hated by peritoneal dialysis have often treated (up to 50 %) of been initially with continuous ultrafiltration or daily haemodialysis. Once fluid balance was improved these patients were then started on peritoneal dialysis [18, 19]. In the acute situation, patients are generally too unfit for general anaesthesia and may be too symptomatic to be able to lie flat for percutaneous insertion of the peritoneal dialysis catheter under local anaesthesia, thus increasing the risks of catheter insertion and malfunction [20]. To overcome rapid transport-induced reduced ultrafiltration, most centres prescribe short peritoneal dialysis cycles, often requiring hypertonic exchanges in combination with 7.5 % icodextrin.

Although peritoneal dialysis may allow patients with pharmacologically refractory CHF to be cared for at home, peritoneal dialysis does not prevent further deterioration in underlying cardiac pathology and as such should be regarded as part of a community-based palliative care package. Short rapid peritoneal dialysis cycles lead to greater water removal than sodium, due to the effect of sodium sieving. 7.5 % icodextrin, which does not have this initial rapid water movement, therefore removes relatively more sodium. In cases of refractory CHF, it may be reasonable to manage patients with two long icodextrin exchanges per day. Although there may be accumulation of the isomaltose polymer, and lead to hyponatremia the life expectancy of these patients is limited, and two icodextrin exchanges per day may reduce the amount of their time spent performing peritoneal dialysis of changes and thus improve their quality of life.

Haemodialysis for the Elderly Patient with Congestive Heart Failure

Vascular Access

Elderly patients with chronic kidney disease and CHF are likely to have vascular calcification. As such, their radial arteries may not be of sufficient internal diameter to successfully create a forearm native arteriovenous fistula. Many surgeons now prefer a two-stage brachial artery fistula, either a brachiocephalic or brachiobasilic anastomosis with subsequent superficialisation of the draining vein. Brachiobasilic fistulae may lead to a vascular steal to the hand. Just as too low a flow through a fistula is undesirable, so is too high a flow for the elderly patient with aortic valve stenosis or other severe valvular heart disease, severe diastolic dysfunction or restrictive cardiomyopathy. The alternative access is the dialysis catheter, and for a patient with limited life expectancy, this may well be the better option.

Choice of Dialyser

As elderly dialysis patients with CHF typically have poor appetite and limited mobility, urea generation rates are lowered, and as such patients can be adequately dialysed with smaller surface area dialysers, without the need to use high blood pump speeds. Dialyser capillary surfaces are negatively charged, and depending upon the charge, when diluted acidic blood from the patient initially flows across the dialyser surface, high-molecular-weight kallikreins are activated, resulting in the generation of bradykinin and complement activation. This reaction can be accelerated by a large bolus of heparin, which contains a series of very negatively charged molecules. Bradykinin is normally very rapidly metabolised, but if patients are prescribed ACEIs for heart failure, then bradykinin clearance is delayed, and patients may suffer hypotensive episodes shortly after starting dialysis. As dialysers differ in the amount of surface charge (zeta potential), use of membranes with less charge or switching ACEIs to ARBs with heparin boluses administered into the venous limb of the extracorporeal circuit (rather than predialyser) may help reduce this anaphylactoid-like reaction.

Choice of Dialysis Schedule

Routine outpatient haemodialysis treatments are often complicated by episodes of intradialytic hypotension. The elderly patient with underlying heart failure is more prone to hypotension, due to changes in central venous capacitance vessels that occur when patients are connected to the extracorporeal circuit. Venodilatation reduced right atrial and ventricular filling pressures and hearts which are stiffer due to diastolic dysfunction are unable to compensate adequately leading to a reduction in left ventricular output and hypotension. Elderly dialysis patients with intrinsic cardiac disease may therefore benefit from more frequent dialysis sessions than the current standard thrice weekly paradigm.

Choice of Ultrafiltration Profile

If the rate of removal of plasma water by dialysis exceeds the vascular refilling rate, hypotension can easily occur, especially in the elderly patient with CHF with already activated sympathetic nervous system and compensatory neurohormonal mechanisms that are soon overwhelmed. Sudden hypotension may lead to cardiac ischaemia. Patients with baseline co-morbidities, including diabetes mellitus, hypertension, CHF, coronary artery disease, dysrhythmia and other cardiac diseases are not only at increased risk of an acute coronary artery syndrome but also more likely to die [21]. As such it is important to reduce the risk of intradialytic hypotension in the elderly dialysis patient with heart failure. Repetitive hypotensive episodes are not only a risk to the heart but also to the brain where, normal autoregulatory defence mechanisms are no longer intact. The risk of ischaemic stroke during hypotensive episodes is much higher in the elderly patient.

Even for healthy patients, an ultrafiltration rate of >10 ml/kg/h is associated with increased risk of hypotension. Therefore, the dialysis sessions may have to be extended to reduce the required ultrafiltration rate [22]. In terms of cardiovascular stability and ultrafiltration rate (UFR), then either a constant UFR or one that starts at a little higher rate followed by a linear decay during dialysis has been observed to cause least hypotension [23].

Choice of Dialysate Electrolyte Composition

During the first hour of dialysis, the serum urea falls exponentially, lowering serum osmolality, that may lead to a reduction in plasma refilling rates and increasing the risk of hypotension. Using a dialysate, sodium concentration higher than plasma will result in a net movement of sodium from the dialysate into the plasma, increasing plasma osmolality and preserve plasma refilling rates despite a falling blood urea level. Even though, raising the dialysate sodium may induce a net positive sodium balance in the patient. . However, since elderly patients with heart failure have reduced appetite and therefore dietary sodium intake, one can afford to use somewhat higher dialysate sodium concentration than those for younger and fitter patients [24].

The risk of hypotension and cardiac arrhythmias can also be reduced by selecting a higher dialysate potassium and calcium concentration. In particular minimising the serum to dialysate potassium gradient to 2.0 mmol/l has been reported to minimise the risk of arrhythmias [25]. In addition low dialysate calcium concentrations of 1 mmol/l increase the risk of cardiovascular instability, and as such higher dialysate calcium concentrations should be chosen [26]. As dietary potassium and calcium intakes are expected to be reduced, then most elderly patients can readily dialyse with higher concentrations; indeed, too, a low serum potassium at the end of the dialysis session is a major risk factor for fatal arrhythmias.

The concentration of bicarbonate in the dialysate is typically set above the normal physiological range, and during haemodialysis the serum bicarbonate rapidly rises. In addition to bicarbonate, a varying amount of acetate is typically present in dialysate concentrates. Supraphysiological bicarbonate dialysates with high acetate concentrations should be avoided as they have been reported to increase the risk of intradialytic hypotension.

Choice of Dialysate Temperature

Closing down capillary beds to skin and pooling of blood in the central venous capacitance vessels increase core body temperature during dialysis, and if the core temperature rises too high, then there will be sudden vasodilatation and hypotension. Thus deliberate cooling of the dialysate will help avoid thermal gains and improve cardiovascular stability [27].

Choice of Dialysis Machine

Dialysis machines differ in their technology to check and regulate dialysate composition and temperature control. Some machines can alter dialysate temperature to prevent thermal heat gain by the patient; others can only provide pre-set temperatures.

More recently several manufacturers have embarked on providing real-time estimation of plasma water as a surrogate for intravascular volume, using either haematocrit or plasma density measurements. Using the relative change in this surrogate for intravascular volume, such dialysis machines with fuzzy logic can regulate dialysate sodium and ultrafiltration rate according to the relative change in relative blood volume. This design may reduce the frequency and severity of intradialytic hypotension [28]. Thus, use of such machines while dialysing elderly patients with CHF seems preferable.

Choice of Dialysis Modality

Although the elderly patient with CHF is unlikely to see any of the longer-term benefits from haemodiafiltration (HDF) compared to standard dialysis, HDF allows an additional cooling effect compared to haemodialysis, particularly in predilutional mode, which may improve cardiovascular instability.

Should Patients Be Given Inotropic Agents to Prevent Intradialytic Hypotension?

Midodrine and to a lesser extent some of the selective serotonin reuptake inhibitors locally increase norepinephrine levels at nerve synapses and have been used to prevent intradialytic hypotension. As these are constrictors, they should be avoided in patients with symptomatic angina. Other centres have infused more potent vasoconstrictors including vasopressin and terlipressin, which may cause digital and gut ischaemia, in addition to coronary artery spasm.

Should Antihypertensive Medications Be Withheld Prior to Dialysis to Prevent Intradialytic Hypotension?

Starting a patient with heart failure on dialysis does not prevent the progression of their underlying heart disease. Since many such medications protect against ischaemia and arrhythmias and improve cardiac remodelling, they should generally not be withheld prior to haemodialysis. Studies of large cohorts of patients have not shown that withholding antihypertensive medications prior to a haemodialysis session reduces the risk of intradialytic hypotension during that session [29].

Summary

Mortality increases with age and co-morbidity, and as such the elderly dialysis patient with congestive heart failure has a shortened life expectancy. Dialysis is only one part of their integrated care package and should be individualised to ensure that the patient can maximise their remaining quality of life. Dialysis prescriptions should primarily be targeted to control extracellular fluid without causing hypotension, rather than primarily focusing on small solute clearance.

Key Points

- Elderly dialysis patients with CHF are at an increased risk of death.
- The distinction between CHF and fluid overload in dialysis patients may be difficult.
- There is a paucity of clear-cut recommendations for the elderly patient with CHF and advanced kidney disease.
- Both haemodialysis and peritoneal dialysis are viable options for dialysis in an elderly patient with CHF.
- Local preference and individual factors may dictate modality choice.
- Adequacy on dialysis in these patients needs some special considerations.
- Peritoneal dialysis has unique advantages of its own besides being a home-based therapy.
- The haemodialysis prescription should be specifically individualised in elderly patients with CHF.
- Dialysis in elderly patients with CHF is only one part of their integrated care package.
- Given high mortality in this patient population, dialysis prescription should specifically focus on controlling excess volume rather than achieving small solute clearances.

References

1. Chan HW, Clayton PA, McDonald SP, Agar JW, Jose MD (2012) Risk factors for dialysis withdrawal: an analysis of the Australia and New Zealand Dialysis and Transplant (ANZDATA) Registry, 1999-2008. Clin J Am Soc Nephrol 7(5):775–781
2. Carson RC, Juszczak M, Davenport A, Burns A (2009) Is maximum conservative management an equivalent treatment option to dialysis for elderly patients with significant comorbid disease? Clin J Am Soc Nephrol 4(10):1611–1619
3. European Society of Cardiology Guidelines for the diagnosis and treatment of acute and chronic heart failure 2012. The Task Force for the Diagnosis and Treatment of Acute and Chronic Heart Failure 2012 of the European Society of Cardiology. Developed in collaboration with the Heart Failure Association (HFA) of the ESC (2012) Eur Heart J 33:1787–1847
4. USRDS annual data report: atlas of chronic kidney disease and end-stage renal disease in the US National Institutes of Health, Diabetes and Digestive and Kidney Diseases 2007, Bethesda
5. Bleyer AJ, Hartman J, Brannon PC, Reeves-Daniel A, Satko SG, Russell G (2006) Characteristics of sudden death in haemodialysis patients. Kidney Int 69:2268–2273
6. CONSENSUS Trial Study Group (1987) Effects of enalapril on mortality in severe congestive heart failure. Results of the Cooperative North Scandinavian Enalapril Survival Study (CONSENSUS). N Engl J Med 316:1429–1435
7. The SOLVD Investigators (1991) Effect of enalapril on survival in patients with reduced left ventricular ejection fractions and congestive heart failure. N Engl J Med 325:293–302
8. Matsumoto Y, Kageyama S, Yakushigawa T, Arihara K, Sugiyama T, Mori Y, Sugiyama H, Ohmura H, Shio N (2009) Long-term low-dose spironolactone therapy is safe in oligoanuric haemodialysis patients. Cardiology 114(1):32–38
9. Asif A, Salman LH, Lopera GG, Carrillo RG (2011) The dilemma of transvenous cardiac rhythm devices in haemodialysis patients: time to consider the epicardial approach? Kidney Int 79(12):1267–1269

10. Winkelmayer WC, Liu J, Setoguchi S, Choudhry NK (2011) Effectiveness and safety of warfarin initiation in older hemodialysis patients with incident atrial fibrillation. Clin J Am Soc Nephrol 6(11):2662–2668

11. Chan KE, Lazarus JM, Thadhani R, Hakim RM (2009) Warfarin use associates with increased risk for stroke in hemodialysis patients with atrial fibrillation. J Am Soc Nephrol 20(10):2223–2233

12. Lip GY, Piotrponikowski P, Andreotti F, Anker SD, Filippatos G, Homma S, Morais J, Pullicino P, Rasmussen LH, Marín F, Lane DA (2012) Thromboembolism and antithrombotic therapy for heart failure in sinus rhythm: an executive summary of a joint consensus document from the ESC Heart Failure Association and the ESC working group on thrombosis. Thromb Haemost 108(6):1009–1022

13. Pamukcu B, Lip GY, Lane DA (2010) Simplifying stroke risk stratification in atrial fibrillation patients: implications of the CHA2DS2-VASc risk stratification scores. Age Ageing 39(5):533–535

14. Fehrman-Ekholm I, Lotsander A, Logan K, Dunge D, Odar-Cederlöf I, Kallner A (2008) Concentrations of vitamin C, vitamin B12 and folic acid in patients treated with haemodialysis and on-line haemodiafiltration or haemofiltration. Scand J Urol Nephrol 42:74–80

15. Cranenburg EC, Schurgers LJ, Uiterwijk HH, Beulens JW, Dalmeijer GW, Westerhuis R, Magdeleyns EJ, Herfs M, Vermeer C, Laverman GD (2012) Vitamin K intake and status are low in haemodialysis patients. Kidney Int 82(5):605–610

16. McKeag NA, McKinley MC, Woodside JV, Harbinson MT, McKeown PP (2012) The role of micronutrients in heart failure. J Acad Nutr Diet 112(6):870–886

17. Sandek A, Bjarnason I, Volk HD, Crane R, Meddings JB, Niebauer J, Kalra PR, Buhner S, Herrmann R, Springer J, Doehner W, von Haehling S, Anker SD, Rauchhaus M (2012) Studies on bacterial endotoxin and intestinal absorption function in patients with chronic heart failure. Int J Cardiol 157(1):80–85

18. Van Der Sande FM, Cnossen TT, Cornelis T, Konings CJ, Kooman JP, Leunissen KM (2012) Peritoneal dialysis in patients with heart failure. Minerva Urol Nefrol 64(3):163–172

19. Nakayama M (2013) Nonuremic indication for peritoneal dialysis for refractory heart failure in cardiorenal syndrome type II: review and perspective. Perit Dial Int 33(1):8–14

20. Cnossen TT, Kooman JP, Krepel HP, Konings CJ, Uszko-Lencer NH, Leunissen KM, van der Sande FM (2012) Prospective study on clinical effects of renal replacement therapy in treatment-resistant congestive heart failure. Nephrol Dial Transplant 27(7):2794–2799

21. Chou MT, Wang JJ, Sun YM, Sheu MJ, Chu CC, Weng SF, Chio CC, Kan WC, Chien CC (2012) Epidemiology and mortality among dialysis patients with acute coronary syndrome: Taiwan National Cohort Study. Int J Cardiol 167(6):2719–2723

22. Saran R, Bragg-Gresham JL, Levin NW, Twardowski ZJ, Wizemann V, Saito A, Kimata N, Gillespie BW, Combe C, Bommer J, Akiba T, Mapes DL, Young EW, Port FK (2006) Longer treatment time and slower ultrafiltration in hemodialysis: associations with reduced mortality in the DOPPS. Kidney Int 69(7):1222–1228

23. Donauer J, Kölblin D, Bek M, Krause A, Böhler J (2000) Ultrafiltration profiling and measurement of relative blood volume as strategies to reduce hemodialysis-related side effects. Am J Kidney Dis 36(1):115–123

24. Shah A, Davenport A (2012) Does a reduction in dialysate sodium improve blood pressure control in haemodialysis patients? Nephrology (Carlton) 17(4):358–363

25. Santoro A, Mancini E, Gaggi R, Cavalcanti S, Severi S, Cagnoli L, Badiali F, Perrone B, London G, Fessy H, Mercadal L, Grandi F (2005) Electrophysiological response to dialysis: the role of dialysate potassium content and profiling. Contrib Nephrol 149:295–305

26. Locatelli F, Covic A, Chazot C, Leunissen K, Luño J, Yaqoob M (2004) Optimal composition of the dialysate, with emphasis on its influence on blood pressure. Nephrol Dial Transplant 19(4):785–796

27. Selby NM, McIntyre CW (2006) A systematic review of the clinical effects of reducing dialysate fluid temperature. Nephrol Dial Transplant 21(7):1883–1898

28. Mancini E, Mambelli E, Irpinia M, Gabrielli D, Cascone C, Conte F, Meneghel G, Cavatorta F, Antonelli A, Villa G, Dal Canton A, Cagnoli L, Aucella F, Fiorini F, Gaggiotti E, Triolo G, Nuzzo V, Santoro A (2007) Prevention of dialysis hypotension episodes using fuzzy logic control system. Nephrol Dial Transplant 22(5):1420–1427
29. Davenport A, Cox C, Thuraisingham R (2008) Achieving blood pressure targets during dialysis improves control but increases intradialytic hypotension. Kidney Int 73(6):759–764

Chapter 13
Dialysis Options for the Elderly Patient with Acute Kidney Injury

Mitchell H. Rosner

Introduction

Acute kidney injury (AKI) is a common and serious event that most often complicates hospitalization for serious illness [1]. Recent data demonstrates that from 2000 to 2009, the incidence of dialysis-requiring AKI increased from 222 to 533 cases per million person-years, an average increase of 10 % per year [2]. An important factor driving this increase in AKI over the past decade is the older age of the population, which serves as an independent risk factor for the development of AKI. It is now clear that the elderly are at the very highest risk for the development of AKI, and over the past 25 years, the mean age of patients with AKI has increased by at least 5 years and perhaps as much as 15 years [3]. In a large European cohort of patients, the average age of patients with AKI was 76 years [4]. Hsu et al. most recently also demonstrated that not only were elderly patients at higher risk for the most severe form of AKI (that requires dialysis) as compared to younger patients, but that over time the incidence of AKI in the elderly is increasing more rapidly than in younger cohorts [2]. At the more severe extremes of AKI, hospitalized patients with dialysis-requiring AKI are older than their counterparts without dialysis-requiring AKI (63.4 versus 47.6 years) [2].

The outcomes for elderly patients who develop dialysis-requiring AKI are uniformly poor with reported mortality rates ranging from 31 to 80 % (with the highest mortality seen in patients requiring dialysis) [5]. In part, the wide variation in these mortality rates is due to study inclusion criteria, differences in whether intensive care unit versus hospital discharge mortality was studied, and definitions for advanced age. Furthermore, in those patients who survive their episode of AKI, an important consideration is the eventual development of chronic kidney disease due

M.H. Rosner, MD
Division of Nephrology, University of Virginia Health System,
Charlottesville, VA, 22908, USA
e-mail: mhr9r@virginia.edu

© Springer Science+Business Media New York 2016
M. Misra (ed.), *Dialysis in Older Adults: A Clinical Handbook*,
DOI 10.1007/978-1-4939-3320-4_13

to the acute insult. Along those lines, in a meta-analysis, Schmitt and co-workers found that patient's age >65 years had significantly worse renal recovery rates as compared with younger patients (31.3 % of surviving elderly patients did not recover kidney function compared with 26 % of younger patients) [6]. Other studies have also demonstrated that the rates of renal recovery after AKI are lower in the elderly [7]. Thus, in those elderly patients who develop dialysis-requiring AKI, the likelihood of renal recovery is lower, leaving patients with the burden of significant CKD and possibly end-stage renal disease (ESRD). This fact is important to consider when making decisions regarding intensive and invasive therapies in elderly patients with multiple comorbid conditions.

Treatment of AKI in the Elderly

There are no specific pharmacological therapies for AKI once it has occurred. Thus, the management of AKI is largely supportive and may include the need for renal replacement support. The decision to initiate renal replacement therapy (RRT) in an elderly patient may be difficult and complex. This decision must factor the possibility that older persons may not fare well on this aggressive, life-sustaining type of therapy and may have competing comorbid conditions that lead to a very poor overall prognosis. Existing outcome data for elderly intensive care unit (ICU) patients requiring dialysis vary widely, with reported mortality ranging from 31 to 80 % [8]. This is due to differences between studies in terms of the definition of advanced age, treatment intensity, severity of illness, and length of follow-up. Some studies report an increased mortality risk in elderly critically ill patients with AKI [8]. Conversely, other well-conducted studies found no difference in mortality attributable to older age (although these studies are older and may not be applicable to current care patterns) [9]. One of these studies found multiple organ dysfunction syndrome (MODS) to be an independent risk factor for increased mortality [10]. Interestingly, those patients with MODS often have a higher acute severity of illness and short-term mortality, but in those who survive, there is lower long-term mortality likely attributable in part to less comorbid illness. Another feature of AKI that has important implications for long-term outcomes is the duration of AKI [11]. In one study, those patients with a duration of AKI greater than 7 days had a higher mortality than those with shorter durations of AKI [11]. Indeed, several studies on long-term outcomes of hospital survivors of MODS and AKI treated with RRT have documented a surprisingly low post-discharge mortality rate and an acceptable self-perceived quality of life [12]. In a multicenter study, Australian New Zealand Care Society Adult Patient (ANCIZS) researchers demonstrated factors associated with lower survival in elderly patients admitted to the ICU [13]. Admission from a chronic care facility, comorbid illness, nonsurgical admission, greater illness severity, mechanical ventilation, and longer stay in ICU were found to be associated with lower patient survival.

Age per se should not be used as criterion to withhold dialysis, and decisions must be individualized accounting for numerous factors, i.e., the severity of illness, likelihood of meaningful physical and cognitive recovery, and family and patient wishes. In this regard, the recent Renal Physicians Association (RPA) guidelines for shared decision making in the appropriate initiation of and withdrawal from dialysis can provide a useful framework for these difficult decisions [14]. In certain circumstances, a time-limited trial of dialysis for those patients with an uncertain prognosis may be warranted. However, all members of the care team and family should agree in advance on the length of the trial as well as the parameters to be assessed during and at the completion of the time-limited trial to determine if dialysis has benefited the patient and whether dialysis should be continued.

There are three critical questions to assess when deciding upon dialysis initiation in the elderly patient with AKI: (1) when to start dialysis and for what indications, (2) what modality of renal replacement therapy should be utilized (intermittent hemodialysis, slow low-efficiency dialysis (SLED), continuous renal replacement or peritoneal dialysis), and (3) how much dialysis is needed or what clearance goals should be prescribed for the patient. In most cases, data specific to the elderly patient are not available, and decisions must be based upon extrapolation of existing data to this population along with expert opinion and the clinician's own experience. It is also important to realize that by the very nature of AKI and its epidemiology, most patients in these studies are greater than age 60 years. The availability of local resources and expertise may also impact decisions.

Initiation of Dialysis in the Elderly Patient with AKI

The traditional indications for this initiation of dialysis in the elderly patient are the same as in other patient groups (Table 13.1). These traditional indications include refractory electrolyte and acid-base disturbances, volume overload refractory to diuretics, and uremic symptoms. However, it is clear that the elderly patient may not tolerate the loss of renal function to the same degree as young patients and thus may develop uremic symptoms, specifically mental status changes, at lower levels of blood urea nitrogen, and therefore, a high index of suspicion must be maintained in assessing for uremic encephalopathy and other uremia-related complications. In cases where uncertainty exists as to whether AKI may be impacting on mental status or other symptoms, a trial of dialysis may be indicated to better assess whether this may be the case.

The timing of initiation of renal replacement therapy for AKI remains a controversial issue with no clear consensus. At the extremes, dialysis initiation could occur only when uremic symptoms and absolute indications (Table 13.1) are present or dialysis could be initiated based upon earlier queues (such as oliguria or specific laboratory levels such as a cutoff value of blood urea nitrogen or creatinine (prophylactic therapy)). In the former case, late dialysis initiation may expose the patient to excessive volume overload or potentially dangerous laboratory values or symptoms. For example, later initiation of dialysis may be associated with increased risk for bleeding; encephalopathy, which increases the risk for aspiration; and limitation of

Table 13.1 Indications for
initiation of dialysis for
patients with acute kidney
injury

Absolute indications:
Hyperkalemia (>6 mEq/L) refractory to medical therapy
Volume overload refractory to diuretic therapy
Azotemia with uremic symptoms
Encephalopathy
Bleeding
Pericarditis
Metabolic acidosis (pH < 7.2) refractory to medical therapy
Other possible indications:
Drug or toxin removal
Removal of contrast agents
Ultrafiltration for volume overload (>10 %)
Hyponatremia in the setting of acute kidney injury or volume overload

nutritional support in an attempt to avoid volume overload and electrolyte abnormalities. On the other hand, earlier prophylactic therapy potentially exposes the patient to an invasive therapy when they might recover renal function with more waiting. The risk here is that the patient may develop a complication associated with dialysis (catheter insertion complications, infection, hemodynamic instability, arrhythmias, and others) when they might have recovered with simply waiting longer. However, complicating this decision-making process is that there are no good predictors on whether a patient with AKI will recover with "watchful waiting" or will progress to absolute indications for dialysis.

Data informing this decision is derived from retrospective cohort studies, observational studies, or the rare, but small and underpowered, randomized controlled trials [15]. Definitions regarding what constitutes early versus late dialysis initiation differ in each study, making conclusions difficult. However, early dialysis generally refers to the start of dialysis based upon decreases in urine output for a short period of time or rises in serum creatinine and/or blood urea nitrogen that are modest in degree. Late dialysis generally refers to the initiation of therapy once clear indications for dialysis are reached or if oliguria is prolonged in duration. A recent systematic review and meta-analysis comparing early versus late initiation of dialysis included 15 studies performed between 1985 and 2010 and calculated an odds ratio for 28-day mortality of 0.45 (95 % confidence interval 0.28–0.72) favoring early initiation of dialysis [16]. However, the authors cautioned that the quality of studies was generally poor. Thus, no clear recommendation for the timing of initiation of dialysis can be offered, and individualized decision making factoring the benefits and risks of early versus late treatment remains the best course of action.

One particular issue of importance when considering the timing of initiation of RRT is the volume status of the patient. Recent data has consistently demonstrated an association of progressive positive fluid balance (>10–20 %) at the time of initiation of RRT with mortality [17]. This data suggests that waiting to start dialysis while the patient is in continued positive fluid balance may be deleterious. However, more data is needed before firm recommendations can be made surrounding the issue of volume balance and initiation of RRT. However, it seems prudent to initiate dialysis if the patient is continuing to experience large positive fluid gains and remains oliguric despite having no specific laboratory indications for initiation.

Selection of Dialysis Modality

Once it is determined that a patient with AKI will require RRT, the clinician must decide upon the modality by which the therapy will be delivered. Broadly speaking, there are two options: (1) conventional intermittent hemodialysis (IHD) and (2) more prolonged therapies which can be delivered continuously (continuous renal replacement therapy (CRRT)) or intermittently but through prolonged sessions (slow low-efficiency dialysis (SLED)). The rationale for utilizing either continuous or more prolonged intermittent therapies rests on the idea that with these treatments, both ultrafiltration and solute removal are slower and thus will minimize the hemodynamic stress in critically ill patients. A comparison of these various therapies is shown in Table 13.2.

Continuous therapies include several subtypes such as continuous venovenous hemofiltration (CVVH), continuous venovenous hemodialysis (CVVHD), and continuous venovenous hemodialfiltration (CVVHDF). The most common indication for choosing a continuous therapy over IHD is the belief that continuous therapies are associated with greater hemodynamic stability. The main determinant of hemodynamic stability during RRT is the maintenance of the intravascular compartment volume. Maintenance of this compartment size rests on slow ultrafiltra-

Table 13.2 Comparison of the techniques available to provide dialysis for the patient with acute kidney injury

	IHD	SLED	CVVH	CVVHD	CVVHDF	PD
Access	VV	VV	VV	VV	VV	PD catheter
Anticoagulation duration	Short	Long	Prolonged	Prolonged	Prolonged	None
BFR (ml/min)	250–400	100–200	200–300	100–200	100–200	N/A
DFR (ml/min)	500–800	100	0	16.7–33.4	16.7–33.4	0.4
Clearance mechanism	Diffusion	Diffusion	Convection	Diffusion	Both	Both
Urea clearance (ml/min)	180–240	75–90	16.7–67	20–30	30–60	8–10
Duration (h)	3–4	8–12	>24	>24	>24	>24

Abbreviations: *IHD* intermittent hemodialysis, *SLED* slow low-efficiency dialysis, *CVVH* continuous venovenous hemofiltration, *CVVHD* continuous venovenous hemodialysis, *CVVHDF* continuous venovenous hemodiafiltration, *BFR* blood flow rate, *DFR* dialysis flow rate, *PD* peritoneal dialysis

tion rates, which allow for movement of fluid from other body compartments into the vascular space to buffer the loss in plasma volume. The other important factor is slow removal of solutes from the intravascular compartment, which lessen the development of a plasma-tissue solute gradient that might favor fluid movement from the vascular to tissue compartments. Continuous therapies, with slower blood flow and dialysate rates as well as with lower ultrafiltration rates, allow for greater maintenance of the intravascular volume. For elderly patients, this may be especially relevant as these patients tend to have higher degrees of hemodynamic instability and due to underlying cardiovascular disease do not tolerate large volume fluid shifts as well as younger patients. Elderly patients are also much more susceptible to the development of delirium which could be exacerbated by rapid solute shifts and changes in intracellular volume. Furthermore, rapid changes in electrolyte levels typically seen with hemodialysis may result in arrhythmias, which would not be well tolerated in the critically ill elderly patient. Whether these theoretical issues translate into improved outcomes with continuous therapies has been a matter of great debate, and no specific comparative data in the elderly population exists.

Numerous studies have tried to compare outcomes among various dialysis modalities [15]. Observational cohort trials are subject to selection bias as those patients receiving continuous therapies are more likely to have had a greater severity of illness and are hemodynamically unstable. Thus, unadjusted mortality rates in observational studies generally show higher mortality rates in the group receiving continuous therapies. When statistical techniques are applied to adjust for baseline differences, the results vary with some studies demonstrating equivalence between intermittent and continuous therapies or finding that one therapy is associated with better outcomes. No consensus results from these studies.

To better elucidate whether intermittent or continuous therapy may be superior, several randomized controlled trials have been attempted. Unfortunately, issues surrounding patient selection and protocol adherence and confounded these studies and has limited their power to discriminate outcomes with different therapies. In those few well-designed and implemented randomized controlled trials, there has been no difference in survival between IHD and CRRT [18, 19]. Furthermore, no trials have demonstrated a difference in the rate of recovery of kidney function between the two modalities [15, 18, 19]. Several meta-analyses and systematic reviews have also not been able to detect an outcome benefit of IHD or CRRT with the exception that CRRT is more effective in leading to negative fluid balance [20, 21]. However, studies have demonstrated that CRRT is a more costly therapy [15, 18–21]. This data set led to the recent Kidney Disease Improving Global Outcomes (KDIGO) Clinical Practice Guidelines for Acute Kidney Injury to recommend viewing CRRT and IHD as complementary therapies with the suggestion to consider the use of CRRT over IHD in hemodynamically unstable patients [22].

Similar to the outcomes between CRRT and IHD, studies between SLED and IHD have not demonstrated that one therapy is superior to another [15]. In many cases, specific institutional limitations may dictate the use of one therapy over another (i.e., CRRT may not be available, and hemodynamically unstable patients may receive SLED instead).

Specific Clinical Situations Favoring the Use of One Form of Dialysis

Patients with increased intracranial pressure (ICP) who develop AKI are at risk for further increases in ICP during IHD. In IHD, rapid diffusion of urea creates a plasma-to-interstitial and interstitium-to-cell osmotic gradient that drives water to the interstitium and to the intracellular compartment. This results in a decrease in plasma volume and cellular edema. The cellular edema within the central nervous system further increases ICP. With CRRT, the slower rate of urea clearance allows for equalization of urea concentrations between compartments and a lower risk of significant fluid shifts between compartments. Thus, with CRRT there is a lower risk of raising ICP, and studies have demonstrated that cerebral perfusion pressure is better maintained with CRRT over IHD [23]. This fact has led to the recommendation to preferentially recommend CRRT for patients with acute brain injury, with cerebral hemorrhage, or with fulminant acute liver failure.

CRRT may also be a preferred option for those patients with severe hyponatremia (serum sodium < 120 meq/L) and AKI [24]. In this case, IHD risks rapid correction of the serum sodium, while CRRT can be prescribed to slowly correct the serum sodium and thus decrease the risk of osmotic demyelination.

Hemodialysis, Hemofiltration, or Hemodiafiltration?

Hemofiltration offers the potential benefit of convective clearance with improved removal of larger molecular weight species (>1000 to 5000 Da). These larger molecular weight species include protein-bound uremic toxins and inflammatory mediators. Theoretically, convective clearance might offer benefit in clinical situations such as sepsis where removal of deleterious cytokines could improve outcomes. However, endogenous production is greater than dialytic removal, and trials have not shown any benefit of hemofiltration over hemodialysis [15]. Thus, there are no conclusive data that favor any one form of solute removal, and as long as adequate overall clearance is adequate, hemofiltration, hemodialysis, and hemodiafiltration are all reasonable options for the provision of CRRT.

Peritoneal Dialysis as an Option for Dialysis of the Patient with AKI

Peritoneal dialysis (PD) has long been used for the treatment of AKI. However, there are few studies that compare outcomes of patients receiving PD versus other modalities. A concern with PD is that clearances tend to be lower than with other forms of dialysis, and thus, for a highly catabolic patient, PD may not provide adequate clearance. Furthermore, there is a risk of PD-associated peritonitis. In one study of patients with falciparum malaria-associated AKI, there was statistically significantly increased mortality as compared with CVVH [25]. However, another study demonstrated similar outcomes between high-volume PD compared to IHD [26]. Available resources often dictate the use of PD as a treatment for AKI, and as with other dialytic therapies, it is critical that adequate clearances be achieved. One advantage of PD over various types of hemodialysis is that there is no need for anticoagulation with PD. However, PD is contraindicated in patients with recent abdominal surgery and may complicate artificial respiratory support due to the changes in intra-abdominal pressure associated with the influx of 2 or more liters of dialysate into the abdominal cavity. Furthermore, for those patients who do not recover renal function after their episode of AKI, rapid conversion to PD ("urgent-start" PD) may offer elderly patients a better method of RRT during their rehabilitation [27]. In this case, PD allows patients to avoid travel to dialysis units, thus maximizing rehabilitation time. Furthermore, the prolonged recovery time after HD is avoided with PD which further increases the ability of the patient to participate in meaningful activity.

What Dose of Dialysis Is Optimum for the Patient with AKI?

Much of the recent research regarding dialysis for the patient with AKI centers on the key question of what is optimum "dose" or clearance that should be provided to patients. In this regard, research has focused on classical clearance of urea and measurement of Kt/Vurea or urea reduction ratio. This excessive focus on urea is due to its convenient measurement and well-established kinetics. However, by focusing solely on urea, the clearance of other potentially important uremic toxins, which may follow different kinetic removal patterns, is neglected. There are no specific studies that assess the dosing of acute dialysis in the elderly population, and it is assumed that patients may respond the same to dosage changes across the spectrum of ages.

In terms of IHD dosing for the patient with AKI, there is only study that examined the benefit of moving from alternate day to daily IHD therapy without changing the intensity of the therapy delivered [28]. This study is confounded by the fact that the daily dose of IHD was suboptimal (Kt/Vurea 0.92–0.94). However, moving from alternate day therapy to daily therapy was associated with a large decrease in mortality. Whether this intensification in the schedule of dialysis would have resulted in the same benefit if an adequate dose of dialysis was given per session is not known.

In the one study investigating extended dialysis (Hanover Dialysis Outcome Study), a total of 156 patients with AKI requiring renal replacement therapy were randomly assigned to receive standard dialysis [dosed to maintain plasma urea levels between 120 and 150 mg/dL] or intensified dialysis [dosed to maintain plasma urea levels <90 mg/dL] [29]. Outcome measures were survival at day 14 (primary) and survival and renal recovery at day 28 (secondary) after initiation of renal replacement therapy. There were no differences in these outcome measures between the groups suggesting that intensification of dialysis dose had no benefit.

Dose calculation for CRRT takes advantage of the fact that there is near-complete equilibration of urea between the blood, dialysate, and ultrafiltrate. Thus, dose calculation is simply derived from the rate of effluent flow (equal to the sum of the dialysate and ultrafiltrate flows) normalized to body weight. This assumes that dialytic and ultrafiltration clearances are equivalent which is an oversimplification. However, for small molecular weight solutes such as urea, this is true.

An initial study assessing the effect of the dose of CRRT on mortality suggested that higher doses were associated with improved outcomes [30]. Patients were randomized to effluent flow rates of 20, 35, or 45 ml/kg/h, and there was an increase in survival measured 15 days after stopping CRRT in the two higher doses of dialysis as compared to the lowest dose (41 % survival with 20 ml/kg/h, 57 % with 35 ml/kg/h, and 58 % with 45 ml/kg/h). A second, larger study assessed the doses of 25 or 40 ml/kg/h of CVVHDF and could not detect a survival difference at 90 days [31]. Another study investigated intensive versus less intensive IHD and CRRT. IHD was provided at a target Kt/V of 1.2–1.4 either six times per week (intensive) or three times per week (less intensive). CRRT was provided either with an effluent flow of 35 ml/kg/h (intensive) or 20 ml/kg/h (less intensive) [32]. In this trial, 60-day all-cause mortality was similar in both groups. Thus, there is no significant benefit associated with more intensive RRT for AKI. Based upon these data, the KDIGO AKI guidelines recommend delivering an effluent volume of 20–25 ml/kg/h for CRRT and a Kt/Vurea of 3.9 per week (equivalent to a dose of 1.2–1.4 three times per week) [22]. In practical terms, it is important to recognize that it is often difficult to achieve the prescribed dose of dialysis for patients with AKI. This is due to the numerous interruptions in therapy that are common in the ICU setting (system clotting, care issues that require interruption in therapy). Thus, it is wise to prescribe a higher dose of dialysis to maintain a buffer to deliver a minimally adequate dose. As in all therapies, an individualized approach is warranted as in some cases higher doses of dialysis may be warranted, such as in a hypercatabolic patient.

Other Issues in the Provision of Dialysis for AKI

Given that one of the most common etiologies of AKI is sepsis, correct dosing of antibiotics is critically important and yet the literature supports the fact that once patients begin dialysis, antibiotics are underdosed and expose the patient to excessive risk from undertreated infections [33]. Whenever possible, drug levels should be followed and maintained at therapeutic levels. If it is not possible to measure drug levels, for those drugs with wide therapeutic indices, it is best to err on the side of higher recommended dosages and closely monitor response to therapy.

Anticoagulation is used to delay or prevent extracorporeal circuit clotting. The two methods utilized to achieve this goal are either intravenous heparin or regional citrate anticoagulation with CRRT [34]. The use of heparin requires close monitoring and is relatively contraindicated in those patients at high risk of bleeding. Regional citrate anticoagulation seems to incur a lower risk of systemic bleeding as compared to heparin since the anticoagulant effects of citrate are largely localized to the extracorporeal circuit. Citrate anticoagulation may lead to metabolic alkalosis as one mmol of citrate is metabolized to bicarbonate. In patients with liver disease, citrate metabolism may be impaired leading to the risk of systemic accumulation of citrate with resulting metabolic acidosis, hypocalcemia, and hypomagnesemia. Thus, when prescribing a citrate-based anticoagulation regime, metabolic monitoring is essential and includes regular assessment of pH, ionized calcium, serum bicarbonate, and sodium and magnesium levels. In those cases where bleeding risk is deemed to be very high, brief use of IHD or CRRT without anticoagulation is possible. With IHD, this requires frequent saline flushes, and with CRRT this can be achieved with prefilter fluid replacement.

Summary

AKI that results in the need for dialysis is associated with a high mortality rate. Elderly patients are at the highest risk for the development of this complication, and decision making in this population may be difficult due to multiple comorbid conditions and uncertainty as to quality of life and the possibility for functional improvement. However, decisions to offer dialysis therapy should not be based solely on age as many elderly patients can achieve significant recovery with supportive care. The past decades have seen tremendous advances in the technology available to provide dialysis support while awaiting renal recovery. However, much uncertainty surrounding the use of these technologies still persists. Fundamental questions such as the proper timing and indications for dialysis, the preferred modality of dialysis support, and the correct dose of dialysis remain without definitive answers. Thus, clinical judgment and individualized assessment and care remain mandatory.

Key Points
1. Acute kidney disease is a common and serious event in the elderly population.
2. Acute kidney disease resulting in the need for renal replacement therapy (RRT) is associated with a high mortality rate, but there is no evidence that older patients fare worse with RRT than younger patients. Thus, decisions regarding the initiation of RRT need to be individualized.
3. The optimal timing for the initiation of RRT is not known, and decisions must balance the risks and benefits of either early or late starts.
4. There is no evidence that one modality of RRT is superior in the therapy of AKI.
5. Patients who are hemodynamically unstable or with evidence of increased intracranial pressure may benefit from continuous renal replacement therapy (CRRT).
6. A minimum dose of RRT must be given to patients with AKI to ensure adequate clearance and volume removal. Doses above this minimal level do not offer additional benefit.

References

1. Lamiere N, Van Biesen W, Vanholder R (2008) Acute kidney injury. Lancet 372:1863–1865
2. Hsu RK, McCulloch CE, Dudley RA et al (2012) Temporal changes in incidence of dialysis-requiring AKI. J Am Soc Nephrol 24:37–42, epub December 6, 2012
3. Turney JH, Marshall DH, Brownjohn AM, Ellis CM, Parsons FM (1990) The evolution of acute renal failure, 1956–1988. Q J Med 74:83–104
4. Ali T, Khan I, Simpson W, Prescott G, Townend J, Smith W et al (2007) Incidence and outcome in acute kidney injury: a comprehensive population-based study. J Am Soc Nephrol 18:1292–1298
5. Chronopoulos A, Rosner MH, Cruz DN, Ronco C (2010) Acute kidney injury in elderly intensive care patients: a review. Intensive Care Med 36:1454–1464
6. Schmitt R, Coca S, Kanbay M et al (2008) Recovery of kidney function after acute kidney injury in the elderly: a systematic review and meta-analysis. Am J Kidney Dis 52:262–271
7. Wald R, Quinn RR, Luo J et al (2009) Chronic dialysis and death among survivors of acute kidney injury requiring dialysis. JAMA 302:1179–1185
8. Uchino S, Kellum JA, Bellomo R et al (2005) Acute renal failure in critically ill patients: a multinational, multicenter study. JAMA 294:813–818
9. Pascual J, Liano F (1998) Causes and prognosis of acute renal failure in the very old. Madrid Acute Renal Failure Study Group. J Am Geriatr Soc 46:721–725
10. Gong Y, Zhang F, Ding F, Gu Y (2012) Elderly patients with acute kidney injury (AKI): clinical features and risk factors for mortality. Arch Gerontol Geriatr 54:e47–e51
11. Coca SG, King JT Jr, Rosenthal RA, Perkal MF, Parikh CR (2010) The duration of postoperative acute kidney injury is an additional parameter predicting long-term survival in diabetic veterans. Kidney Int 78:926–933
12. Morgera S, Kraft AK, Siebert G, Luft FC, Neumayer HH (2002) Long-term outcomes in acute renal failure patients treated with continuous renal replacement therapies. Am J Kidney Dis 40:275–279
13. de Mendonca A, Vincent JL, Suter PM et al (2000) Acute renal failure in the ICU: risk factors and outcome evaluated by the SOFA score. Intensive Care Med 26:915–921
14. Renal physician association shared decision making in the appropriate initiation of and withdrawal from dialysis, 2nd ed. Available at: http://www.renalmd.org/catalogue-item.aspx?id=682. Accessed 30 Jan 2013
15. Palevsky P (2013) Renal replacement therapy in acute kidney injury. Adv Chronic Kid Dis 20:76–84
16. Karvellas CJ, Farhat MR, Sajjad I et al (2011) A comparison of early versus late initiation of renal replacement therapy in critically ill patients with acute kidney injury: a systematic review and meta-analysis. Crit Care 15:R72
17. Bouchard J, Sorroko SB, Chertow GM et al (2009) Fluid accumulation, survival and recovery of kidney function in critically ill patients with acute kidney injury. Kidney Int 76:422–427
18. Lins RL, Elseviers MM, Ven de Niepen P et al (2009) Intermittent versus continuous renal replacement therapy for acute kidney injury patients admitted to the intensive care unit: results of a randomized clinical trial. Nephrol Dial Transplant 24:512–518
19. Vinsonneau C, Camus C, Combes A et al (2006) Continuous venovenous hemodiafiltration versus intermittent hemodialysis for acute renal failure in patients with multiple-organ dysfunction syndrome : a multicenter randomized trial. Lancet 368:379–385
20. Rabindranath K, Adams J, Macleod AM, Muirhead N (2007) Intermittent versus continuous renal replacement therapy for acute renal failure in adults. Cochrane Database Syst Rev 3, CD003773
21. Bagshaw SM, Berthiaume LR, Delancy A, Bellomo R (2008) Continuous versus intermittent renal replacement therapy for critically ill patients with acute kidney injury: a meta-analysis. Crit Care Med 36:610–617

22. Group KDIGOKAKIW (2012) KDIGO clinical practice guidelines for acute kidney injury. Kidney Int Suppl 2:1–138
23. Davenport A (2009) Continuous renal replacement therapies in patients with acute neurological injury. Semin Dial 22:165–168
24. Lenk MR, Kaspar M (2012) Sodium-reduced continuous venovenous hemodiafiltration (CVVHDF) for the prevention of central pontine myelinolysis (CPM) in hyponatremic patients scheduled for orthotopic liver transplantation. J Clin Anesth 24:407–411
25. Phu NH, Hien TT, Mai NY et al (2002) Hemofiltration and peritoneal dialysis in infection-associated acute renal failure in Vietnam. N Engl J Med 347:895–902
26. Gabriel DP, Caramori JT, Martin LC et al (2009) Continuous peritoneal dialysis compared with daily hemodialysis in patients with acute kidney injury. Perit Dial Int 29(Suppl 2): S62–S71
27. Ghaffari A (2012) Urgent-start peritoneal dialysis: a quality improvement report. Am J Kidney Dis 59:400–408
28. Schiffl H, Lang SM, Fischer R (2002) Daily hemodialysis and the outcome of acute renal failure. N Engl J Med 346:305–310
29. Faulhaber-Walter R, Hafer C, Jahr N et al (2009) The Hannover Dialysis Outcome Study: comparison of standard versus intensified extended dialysis for treatment of patients with acute kidney injury in the intensive care unit. Nephrol Dial Transplant 24:2179–2186
30. Ronco C, Bellomo R, Homel P et al (2000) Effects of different doses in continuous venovenous hemofiltration on outcomes of acute renal failure: a prospective randomized trial. Lancet 356:26–30
31. Bellomo R, Cass A, Cole L et al (2009) Intensity of continuous renal replacement therapy in critically ill patients. N Engl J Med 361:1627–1638
32. Palevsky PM, Zhng JH, O'Connor TZ et al (2008) Intensity of renal support in critically ill patients with acute kidney injury. N Engl J Med 359:7–20
33. Fissell WH (2013) Antimicrobial dosing in acute renal replacement. Adv Chronic Kidney Dis 20:85–93
34. Davenport A, Mehta S (2002) The acute dialysis quality initiative- part VI. Access and anticoagulation in CRRT. Adv Renal Replace Ther 9:273–281

Chapter 14
Dialysis Versus Conservative Care in the Elderly: Making a Choice

Aine Burns

Introduction

The aging process results in marked alterations in the kidneys, impairing their ability to maintain homeostasis, adapt to changing local environments and recover from injury. These changes are both anatomical and functional and have been considered the cause of the increased propensity of the elderly to acute or chronic renal failure that may be accelerated and/or accentuated by diseases such as diabetes mellitus and hypertension.

Frailty is a biologic syndrome of decreased reserve, and resistance to stressors that results from cumulative decline across multiple physiologic systems is common in elderly CKD patients. Protein-energy wasting (PEW), sarcopenia, dynapenia, etc., which accompany frailty, contribute to poor outcomes.

One of the biggest challenges nephrologists face is how to best serve frail elderly and (increasingly) very elderly patients who present with advanced CKD.

Perhaps the most important thing to recognise from the outset is that each individual patient presents with his or her own unique set of social, medical and cognitive as well ethical and moral circumstances requiring multiple and individually tailored solutions.

A further consideration is the changing nature of this field as populations survive even longer and patient and public expectations adjust accordingly. Arguably, nephrology has become the victim of its own success as renal replacement therapy has become technically possible even in the sickest patients [1].

Yet, despite anecdotal success stories, there are numerous elderly people for whom dialysis has not been a success, where symptom burden and quality of life is

A. Burns, MB, BaO, Bch, MRCPI, MD, FRCP, MSc Med Ed
Department of Medicine, Centre for Nephrology, University College London,
Royal Free NHS Foundation Trust, London, UK
e-mail: aine.burns@nhs.net

© Springer Science+Business Media New York 2016
M. Misra (ed.), *Dialysis in Older Adults: A Clinical Handbook*,
DOI 10.1007/978-1-4939-3320-4_14

poor and death may even have been hastened and certainly medicalised. The number of patients withdrawing from dialysis programmes bears witness to this fact. These latter considerations have led many clinicians to offer a structured alternative 'conservative or supportive care' to elderly patients with advanced CKD. In recent years, the success of these endeavours has enshrined 'conservative care' (CC) as a legitimate alternative to haemo- or peritoneal dialysis, particularly for the frail older patient. This chapter will explore the current evidence clinicians can draw upon to help inform an individual patient's choice and deliver optimal non-dialytic or conservative care (CC).

Historical Perspective

Since the introduction of chronic dialysis in the 1960s, there has been increasing demand fuelled by technical success, medical advances and increased patient and public expectation. In the early years of chronic dialysis, treatment was unashamedly rationed with young, otherwise healthy, candidates, or those with dependent families being chosen amongst the lucky few to receive treatment! Throughout the 1980s and 1990s, increasingly older patients were commenced on dialysis, many with very significant additional co-morbidity. Crude survival amongst these patients was shockingly poor: as bad or even worse than many advanced cancers. Furthermore, these patients were found to suffer a considerable burden of physical symptoms [2], and many authors reported a marked and permanent deterioration in functional status and quality of life (QOL) after dialysis initiation [3]. Thus, many nephrologists have questioned the wisdom of offering dialysis to all comers. It has been suggested that a conservative approach might be a more humane way to deal with advanced CKD in elderly patients, particularly in those with poor functional status and multiple other co-morbidities. Over the past decade, there has been a growing wave of interest in CC both in palliative and geriatric care communities and amongst nephrologists [4, 5]. Conservative and end-of-life care together with symptom management are now included on the curriculum for nephrology trainees on both sides of the Atlantic. Today, most renal units in the developed world aspire to deliver symptom-driven multidisciplinary care to their elderly patients with an increasing realisation that the removal of waste solute and water, alone, is not the answer. In recent years, the take-on rates for dialysis programmes have plateaued in many European countries. However, it is not known what part the emergence of CC has played in this change.

Terminology for Non-dialytic Management

There is no consensus regarding terminology for these latter approaches. Table 14.1 outlines the commonly used terms. For the purposes of this chapter, we will use the term conservative care (CC).

Table 14.1 Terms used for non-dialytic conservative therapies

Conservative management
Conservative care
Maximum conservative management
Renal supportive care
Residual renal support
Palliative renal care
Conservative kidney care
The non-dialysis option
Structured supportive care

This varied terminology reflects significant differences in approaches to care for patients who either do not wish to receive dialysis or are deemed not suitable and therefore are not offered renal replacement therapy. Treatment pathways vary as well. On one hand, patients may be discharged back into the community with no renal follow-up with the label 'unsuitable for dialysis'. On the other hand, intensive patient and family education regarding treatment options, prognosis and complications are offered with shared decision-making and follow-up by renal services. Such programmes usually include anaemia management, symptom control, treatment of intercurrent illnesses and a package of social and supportive services that can be escalated as the patient's condition deteriorates. Some programmes also strongly encourage patients to create advance directives or other formal end-of-life plans.

The existing terminology does not define whether a plan for CC was initiated by the patient alone, with their families or on the recommendation of a nephrologist or other health professional. Very few registries exist to catalogue CC patient outcomes. Similarly, the motivation behind CC decisions is rarely recorded and has only been investigated in a handful of very small studies.

Dialysis Choices

The choice of dialysis treatments for elderly patients has broadened in recent years. Regular haemodialysis (HD) is performed for the most part in the same manner as for younger patients. Conventional peritoneal dialysis (PD) performed four times daily by the patient or a family member at home can now be replaced by overnight or automated peritoneal dialysis (APD) systems and more recently, in some countries, by assisted peritoneal dialysis (see chapter on PD).

Conservative Care Versus Dialysis

Dialysis places a significant burden on elderly patients, their families and health service. There is evidence that elderly HD patients experience an increased rate of deterioration in functional and mental capacity on haemodialysis and have a symptom burden and quality of life comparable to patients with advanced cancer. By contrast, many patients who choose a CC approach appear to have a fairly flat functional trajectory until a short time before death. Symptom burden in both groups has been shown to be high and may not differ significantly between patients undergoing dialysis and CC. Yet, impressive survivals have been documented in both cohorts of patients who commenced dialysis over the age of 80 years [6] or followed CC programmes [4].

Trajectories of decline in renal function vary hugely and often unpredictably with many elderly patients having a very slow decline and surviving with minimal (<5 ml/min) measured creatinine clearance. Thus, the boundaries are unclear as to when dialysis confers overall benefit. There are no controlled trials of CC versus dialysis, but several authors have attempted to determine whether dialysis significantly prolongs life in the old and frail. Current evidence suggests that although dialysis may extend survival, the number of out-of-hospital intervention-free days does not differ much between the two groups [7] and the survival benefit disappears as co-morbidity increases and functional status declines [4]. A convincing argument in favour of CC in patients over the age of 80 with high co-morbidity or poor functional status purely on the grounds of survival benefit has been put forth [8]. CC patients are also more likely to die at home or in a hospice than in an acute hospital setting. It is not clear whether dialysis improves symptoms or quality of life or merely exchanges one set of symptoms for another in the frail and elderly. Given the same education and free choice, older frailer patients choose CC [9]. Interestingly, there is also some evidence to suggest that survival curves diverge between groups of patients who choose CC compared with dialysis at relatively high e-GFRs, i.e. well before dialysis is initiated.

Symptom Prevalence in CC Patients

Elderly patients with advanced CKD and multiple co-morbidities have been shown to have high symptom and depression scores in cross-sectional studies. However, little is known about symptom trajectory over time and the effect of interventions such as dialysis. Detailed measurements of symptom burden are cumbersome and impractical for routine use in all patients. Table 14.2 reports the symptom prevalence in a cohort of CC UK patients [2].

Survival and Quality of Life

There are no randomised trials to determine whether elderly patients who choose dialysis over CC survive longer. It is unlikely that such studies will be undertaken for ethical reasons. However, there are several studies that catalogue the outcomes of elderly and very elderly patients on dialysis. Very impressive survival (median survival 46.5 months, range 0–107) has been reported by some for those who

Table 14.2 Symptom Prevalence in Conservatively Managed CKD patients [2]

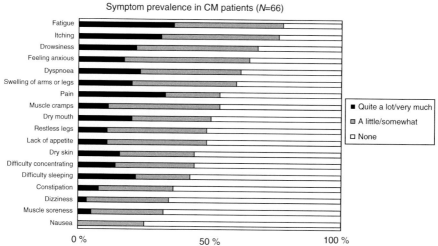

initiated dialysis in their eight decade [6]. Registry data, however, would suggest that elderly people, particularly those with poor functional status and multiple co-morbidities, fare poorly with very many surviving less than 6 months on dialysis. A few studies have compared survival between patients undergoing dialysis and CC [4]. However, all studies are flawed by possible selection bias of healthier younger patients for dialysis intervention. Many authors have questioned whether such dialysis interventions are merely prolonging dying rather than extending meaningful life. Carson et al. who retrospectively examined survival and hospitalisation in a single unit's population of over 75 year olds found an increased survival in those dialysed but reported that almost every day of life gained was at the expense of a day spent in a hospital environment either on dialysis or as an inpatient [7]. Murtagh et al. reported that 1- and 2-year survival rates were 84 and 76 % in a group of patients opting for dialysis ($n=52$) and 68 and 47 % in those on a CC pathway ($n=77$) [10]. However, the survival advantage was lost in those patients with high co-morbidity scores, especially when ischemic heart disease was present. Da-Silva has recently reported that CC patients in their unit were older, more dependent and more highly co-morbid, had poorer physical health and higher anxiety levels than those choosing dialysis. Mental health, depression and life satisfaction scores were similar even when examined longitudinally. They also demonstrated that quality-of-life measures except life satisfaction decreased significantly after dialysis initiation but remained stable in CC patients. Their model, which controlled for co-morbidity, Karnofsky performance scale, age, physical health score and propensity score, con-firmed an increased survival in HD patients (median survival from recruitment: 1317 days in HD patients (mean of 326 dialysis sessions) and 913 days in CC patients). Therefore, they concluded that patients choosing CC did not live as long as their counterparts on dialysis but maintained a better quality of life. Adjusted median survival from recruitment was 13 months shorter for CC patients than HD patients [9]. Likewise, Hussain found a survival advantage for their patients who chose dialysis over CC, but this disappeared in the older frailer patients [8]. Whether post-dialysis initiation rehabilitation interventions would improve quality of life or longevity in this elderly co-morbid group is not known.

The Trajectory of Illness

Distinct trajectories of illness over time and towards death are well described in many diseases. Understanding these trajectories can facilitate standard of care and optimal timing of discussions about goals of care, symptom management and advance care planning in the last months of life. A different functional trajectory over the last year of life has been described in CC renal patients (Table 14.3). This is likely to help facilitate best timing and configuration of care.

On average, CC patients report low to moderate levels of physical and psychological symptom distress through the course of their illness. However, they report increasing concerns about the need for information as the duration of illness extends. CC patients also experience a marked increase in symptoms and quite sudden decline in functional status in the last weeks of life. Worsening symptoms may be a much better prognostic indicator than biochemical or other disease markers [11].

However, this 'average' trajectory, which is helpful for service development and planning, does not always reflect the patterns for an individual patient. Amongst CC patients, three discrete symptom trajectories have emerged: (1) relatively stable, (2) steadily increasing and (3) markedly fluctuant, with this pattern occurring more often in those with concurrent cardiac and/or respiratory disease. This latter fluctuant and unpredictable pattern is associated with much higher psychological distress amongst patients and families coping with recurrent acute crises with uncertain outcome. Several investigators have identified that 1–2 weeks prior to death CC patients experience an increase in symptoms. This has been termed the 'tipping point' or transition and is where interventions to address symptoms and other concerns can be targeted to provide most benefit. Further research and a better understanding of illness trajectories in CC and end-stage kidney disease are needed.

Table 14.3 Functional Trajectory Using Karnofsky Performance Scores (KPS) in the last year of life of Conservatively Managed CKD Patients= Left hand side, Recognized Functional Trajectories in various other conditions =Right hand side [11]

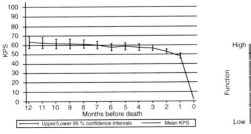 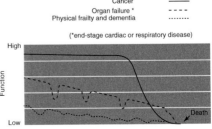

Delivering Conservative Care

Once a decision has been made to follow a CC pathway, the emphasis of care should shift from preparation for renal replacement therapy to symptom control, maintenance of residual renal function, avoiding acute medical events likely to destabilise the patient's condition and minimising complications related to CKD. Reversible causes of CKD need to be considered and treated where possible and constant attention paid to minimise pill burden.

Symptom Control

The prevalence and variety of patient reported symptoms is now well recognised. In untreated or newly referred patients, many relate to anaemia and most units are adept at improving and maintaining haemoglobin (Hb) using both iron and subcutaneously administered erythroid-stimulating agents (ESAs) with only occasional need for transfusion. Protocols vary from unit to unit, but in general the availability of erythropoietin and safe intravenous iron preparations have meant that Hb can be maintained at target levels in the majority. In general, target Hb are those used in the dialysis population. Maintenance of Hb has the added advantage of mitigating some of the distress caused by angina and CHF and can improve physical functioning and fatiguability.

Longer-acting ESAs are particularly useful in elderly patients especially if community nurses are required to administer the injections.

Several studies confirm the high prevalence of pain in HD and CKD patients opting for CC. In general NSAIDs are harmful to residual kidney function and may cause or exacerbate GI haemorrhage. Other analgesics, particularly opiates, accumulate or are metabolised differently in advanced CKD [12]. This issue is discussed at length later in this chapter. Hence, caution needs to be exercised to eliminate pain without causing additional problems.

Preserving Residual Function

When supporting residual renal function in elderly CKD patients, clinicians should have several objectives: perhaps the most important is pre-empting and avoiding intercurrent illnesses that can precipitate acute deterioration. In men, care should be taken to consider and treat new or worsening bladder outflow obstruction that might be silently accelerating decline in renal function. Minimising proteinuria and optimising blood pressure and glycaemic control in diabetics are desirable but may not markedly slow progression in this group. In such vulnerable patients, it is often wise to accept trade-offs between optimal control of blood sugar and BP and potential problems created by the tools used to achieve them. Thus, for individual patients the clinician may need to be pragmatic in their interpretation of guidelines and targets designed for younger and fitter patients. Use of angiotensin-converting enzyme inhibitors (ACEIs) or angiotensin receptor blockers (ARBs) to control both BP and reduce proteinuria is desirable but should be instituted with a close watch on renal function and worsening hyperkalaemia. In practice, if potassium control is difficult, it may be necessary to discontinue them. Discontinuing ACEI or ARBs may have the added benefit of 'buying back' a few mls of residual renal clearance. This strategy has been examined by Goncalves et al. who concluded by questioning the universal pre-emptive initiation of RAS inhibitors in advanced CKD and suggested that they could be safely stopped, at least in some patients particularly those on CC pathways [13]. Caution needs to be exercised, however, if cardio-renal syndrome is present. Whether optimising Hb prolongs residual renal function is not known.

Managing Diet, Nutrition and Fluid Balance

In the era before chronic dialysis became widely available, clinicians advised draconian dietary restrictions to control intake of protein, potassium and phosphate in CKD to extend survival. However, the cost to the patient was often severe malnutrition with profound muscle wasting. In contrast, most CC programmes now emphasise maintenance of a low-salt, normal-protein diet, encouraging patients to eat and enjoy the foods they like, in order to maintain flesh weight and enhance quality of life (QOL). If hyperkalaemia or hyperphosphotaemia becomes problematic, limited dietary restrictions may be appropriate. However, it is important to remain mindful of the important part food contributes towards optimising QOL which underpins the ethos of CC. In reality, elderly and frail CKD patients often lose enjoyment of food as CKD progresses, and renal dieticians need to be creative in augmenting diets rather than restricting them. Food supplements can be used to good effect in some patients.

Controlling phosphate by dietary or pharmacological means may help reduce the distressing symptom of itch. Some authors suggest that optimal Ca and phosphate control slows progression of CKD. However, a balance needs to be established between the potential benefits of phosphate control and the negative effects of dietary restriction and increasing the pill burden in CC patients. Aggressive avoidance or treatment of hyperparathyroidism is only relevant, in this group, if there are symptoms such as bone pain or fractures or as a part of the efforts to alleviate itch. There is some data suggesting that treating hyperparathyroidism, per se, impacts overall survival in CKD patients, but once again the clinician has to judge the relevance of treating a patient with very limited life expectancy. Similarly, many clinicians actively seek to identify and treat reduced vitamin D levels, yet, despite a glut of recent publications concerning ESRD patients, it is not known whether this is advantageous in CC patients.

Finally, many CKD patients erroneously believe that increased fluid intake will 'help' their kidneys to 'work better'. Others have particular difficulty excreting salt and water because of either concurrent diabetic nephropathy or heart failure. Advice about fluid intake therefore needs to be individualised depending on the particular circumstances pertaining to the patient. Many if not most elderly patients with advanced CKD require diuretics. Loop diuretics are the most commonly prescribed. They can however cause AKI in addition to the existing CKD and exacerbate urinary frequency, nocturia and gout. Consequently, once again, their dose and timing needs to be considered carefully on an individual basis.

Minimising Futile Interventions

If possible, clinicians should clarify, in advance, whether a CC patient wishes to receive dialysis for a limited time to overcome a temporary reduction in renal function that might, for example, result from an intercurrent respiratory tract or other infection. Similarly, 'ceilings of care' in accordance with a patient's wishes may be usefully discussed and documented. Formalised advanced care plans or directives can be helpful and are in general desirable, although uptake of this option where formally offered is low (author's personal experience).

Decision-Making

Decision-making about ESRD is often/always challenging for elderly patients, their families and professionals. There is limited evidence to guide practice. Most people tend to focus on living rather than dying. CKD patients can become accustomed to living with their chronic conditions, and many patients, their families and even their clinicians are reluctant to consider the implications of future deterioration. Others are focussed on their additional co-morbid conditions and can be unaware of the severity and implications of their renal disease. However, based on the small amount of evidence available, important points that elderly patients who choose CC consider in reaching their decision include avoiding poor quality of life, minimising pain and suffering, a desire not to be a burden to care givers, feeling 'too old' for dialysis and that it would be more 'natural' to die without dialysis and not wishing to attend the hospital frequently [14]. Discrete choice experiments in Australian patients suggest that travel restrictions are an important additional consideration and that patients were willing to forgo a surprisingly long duration of life expectancy (23 months, 95 % CI, 19–27) in order to decrease the travel restrictions that dialysis would impose [15]. In general, however, the processes and determinants of decisions for or against the CC are poorly understood. Preserved cognitive function, particularly higher mental function, is clearly an important consideration when appraising patients of treatment options and facilitating informed choice. A proactive and open approach towards decision-making is recommended, but is difficult to achieve. A recent web-based survey of nephrologists in Europe found that nephrologists decided to offer CC in 5–20 % of patients and a further 5 % of patients chose CC as they refused when nephrologists intended for them to start dialysis [16].

Timely Communication and Advance Care Planning

The importance of timely information, which meets individual patients' preferences, cannot be overstated. Patients with advanced CKD may have been receiving nephrology care for some months or years and become used to living with their renal disease. Thus, it can be difficult for professionals to open up conversations about deterioration or decline in health, and limited survival, when these begin to become relevant. Delivery of optimal palliative and supportive care for patients starts with honest prognostic information, tailored to the patient's information preferences. Many factors prevent good communication, including the inherent uncertainty of prognostication, the uncertainty of an individual trajectory of illness, the imbalance of knowledge between patients and professionals, cognitive impairment and the perceived and actual time limitations in busy health care settings.

The annual mortality rate of dialysis patients approaches 20–24 %. This is higher than that of prostate, breast or colorectal cancer, but many renal patients and their families are not aware of this and consider renal failure as curable with transplantation or treatable with dialysis. Open prognostic information to counter this should be offered even before treatment pathways are considered, but this occurs infrequently.

Advance care planning is a dynamic process that does not occur at one point in time. A good relationship with the patient, and an understanding of their perspectives, is important before having discussions about future priorities and preferences for care. Palliative and supportive care emphasises improving quality of life as end-of-life approaches, and this can only be achieved if there is genuine communication as a foundation for planning, considering outstanding issues and addressing family relationships and conflict. Davison, when studying advanced care planning, showed that patients wanted more information and, in non-medical language on prognosis, disease process and the impact of treatment on daily life [17].

Renal professionals often need prompts to help them open up discussion about the future, as they are much less familiar with how to do this than palliative care professionals. But when sensitive, open exploration of concerns for the future is achieved, the discussion is usually appreciated by patients [18].

Symptom Assessment

Symptom alleviation in renal failure patients is very challenging for many reasons. The symptoms commonly go unrecognised, and renal impairment may constrain management with drugs. It is not always clear whether uraemia or co-morbid

Table 14.4 Symptom
assessment scoring systems
for renal patients

Edmonton Symptom Assessment System
Memorial Symptom Assessment Scale
The Dialysis Symptom Index
The renal version of the Patient Outcome Scale
The distress thermometer*
Individual symptom scoring systems (pain, depression, pruritus, restless legs syndrome)

*Data only published in abstract form at the time of going
to press

conditions are the main cause of each symptom, and for many patients, a combination of factors contributes to their overall symptom burden. The diabetic patient poses particular challenges in this regard and illustrates the difficulties. Diabetic gastroparesis is characterised by anorexia, early satiety, nausea and sometimes vomiting. Advanced uraemia itself also leads to delayed gastric emptying, gastric reflux and dyspepsia. Additional autonomic nerve damage affecting the mid- and lower gut may cause alternating diarrhoea and constipation. Neuropathic pain can be severe, persistent and difficult to control. Skin and soft tissue problems are also common; decubitus ulcers or diabetic foot may occur and amputation may sometimes be required. In these circumstances, clinical judgement skills are critical if complex diagnostic interventions are to be avoided and symptom alleviation maximised which can be helpful (Table 14.4).

A variety of symptom assessment scoring systems have been developed or validated for or used in groups of renal patients. They vary from the long and in-depth memorial symptom assessment score where 32 symptoms are scored for frequency, severity and impact to the simple distress thermometer validated and used widely in cancer services.

Management of Common Symptoms

Pain

Pain is such a common yet under-recognised and under-treated finding in elderly renal patients, and it deserves special attention.

Firstly, removal or specific treatment of the underlying cause of pain is (when feasible) always the best approach, and only when this cannot be achieved should palliation be the main focus. Non-opioid, opioid and adjuvant analgesics can be used in CC patients, but it is critically important not to risk remaining renal function, and careful consideration must be paid to altered metabolism and excretion in the context of renal impairment to avoid unnecessary adverse events.

There are reports of serious side effects following codeine and dihydrocodeine use in patients with advanced renal failure, in particular profound hypotension, respiratory arrest and narcolepsy. For these reasons, they are not recommended.

90 % of tramadol is excreted via the kidneys, resulting in a twofold increase in the elimination half-life in renal impairment; therefore, the dose interval should be increased to twelve hourly, and the dose reduced. Uraemia also lowers the seizure threshold, and tramadol may be more epileptogenic in CC patients.

Morphine and diamorphine are not recommended, because of problems with metabolite accumulation, some of which are clinically active.

Less than 10 % of fentanyl is excreted unchanged in the urine. In renal failure, no dose modification appears necessary. One study however suggests accumulation with sustained administration, and a further study demonstrates reduced clearance. Despite these concerns, fentanyl is, on present limited evidence, one of the preferred opioids in CC patients, and the metabolites are inactive. Some authorities suggest 50 % normal dose if creatinine clearance is <10 ml/min. Careful monitoring for any gradual development of accumulation and toxicity is advised with sustained administration (beyond 1 or 2 days), and there may be some basis for gradual dose reduction if fentanyl is used over days or weeks. Transdermal patches make administration easy. However, a wide individual variation in the pharmacokinetics of fentanyl has been observed and supports a cautious approach.

Alfentanil is shorter acting than fentanyl, but is limited to very end-of-life use as it is only available parenterally.

Buprenorphine because of its high systemic clearance and largely hepatic metabolism has the potential to be reasonably safe in CC patients. Some evidence shows no change in the pharmacokinetics of buprenorphine in renal impairment, but other work shows accumulation of metabolites, although adverse effects have not been reported. Buprenorphine also has the advantage of being available in sublingual, transdermal and injectable preparations (12 Murtagh 2007).

Hydromorphone is likely to accumulate in renal impairment (with proportionately greater accumulation in more severe renal impairment), and clear guidance on its use cannot be given until there is more evidence available.

Methadone is metabolised mostly in the liver and excreted both renally and faecally. There is large interindividual variation and also considerable difference between acute and chronic phase metabolism. Caution should be exercised, and experienced specialist supervision of methadone is required, making it a less valuable tool in CC patients.

Elimination of oxycodone and its metabolites in renal failure is significantly prolonged. There is insufficient evidence to determine whether or not it is safe to use in ESRD patients. Some clinicians use it with caution by reducing the dose and increasing the dosing interval.

Fatigue

Fatigue is multidimensional, with physical, cognitive and emotional elements. Sleep disturbance, poor physical functioning and depression commonly accompanying renal disease may contribute. A number of causes are potentially treatable.

These may be related to the renal disease, e.g. anaemia, or to co-morbid conditions, e.g. hypothyroidism or heart failure, and should be treated aggressively. There is a consistent relationship between haematocrit and energy/fatigue domains in health-related quality of life scores. So for CC patients also, maintenance of Hb is paramount. Non-pharmacological managements of fatigue, such as exercise, cognitive and psychological approaches and complementary treatments, are important, especially as pharmacological interventions become increasingly limited [19].

Nausea and Vomiting

Nausea and vomiting are extremely unpleasant symptoms and are often multifactorial. The first step is to identify any specific cause if present, since cause-directed treatment is most likely to succeed. Uraemia, drugs, gastroparesis or delayed gastric emptying should all be considered. Constipation may exacerbate nausea and vomiting. Poor and/or erratic absorption of oral medications may result, and alternative routes (sublingual, rectal or subcutaneous) need to be considered.

Metoclopramide can be used for delayed gastric emptying or gastroparesis, although doses should be reduced by 50 %, for severe renal impairment. There is also an increased risk of dystonia. Haloperidol or levomepromazine is often used for nausea related to uraemia or drugs, although due to increased cerebral sensitivity, both drugs need dose reduction. 5HT3 antagonists can also be used, although the side effect of constipation needs active management. Because gastritis is common amongst uraemic patients, a low threshold for treatment with a proton pump inhibitor is advised if gastritis is a contributory factor.

Pruritus

The aetiology and pathogenesis of pruritus in ESRD remain unclear, and treatment is frustratingly suboptimal. Current explanatory hypotheses postulate abnormal inflammatory/immune processes, dysfunction in the opioid receptor system and/or neuropathic processes within the nervous system itself.

Thus, immune modulators (such as ultraviolet B light, tacrolimus and thalidomide), opioids antagonists such as naloxone and naltrexone, a relatively new κ-opioid agonist nalfurafine, neuropathic agents (lidocaine, gabapentin) and capsaicin as a counterirritant have all been trialled to treat itch, with varying success. The most commonly used agents, antihistamines, often fail to resolve the itch, but most practitioners would suggest them before moving on to other agents. An important factor in ESRD-related itch is xerosis, or dry skin, that may be a particularly important factor in older people and should be countered with generous and frequent application of emollients. Other common causes of pruritus such as skin disorders; skin infections, e.g. scabies; and liver impairment, especially if the symptom is not resolving, need to be considered.

The first management step is to optimise phosphate levels which contribute significantly to pruritus. Hyperparathyroidism may also be a factor and should be considered. Older people living alone may find it difficult to apply emollients, and spray applications can be helpful in this instance. Preventive measures, such as nail care (keeping nails short), keeping cool (light clothing) and tepid baths or showers are useful concurrent measures. The psychological and social dimensions of severe itch are considerable, and psychological, family and social support is an important component of management [20].

Restless Legs

Restless legs syndrome (RLS) is characterised by uncomfortable sensation and/or an urge to move the legs, worsening at rest, especially during the night. It is often partially or totally relieved by physical activity. The exact cause is not well understood, but the dopaminergic neurons, in the central nervous system, are thought to be disrupted. Iron deficiency, low parathyroid hormone levels, hyperphosphataemia and psychological factors may all play a role. Treatment should involve correction of these factors and reduction of potential exacerbating agents, such as caffeine, alcohol and nicotine. Drugs including sedative antihistamines, metoclopramide, tricyclic antidepressants, selective serotonin uptake inhibitors, lithium, dopamine antagonists and calcium antagonists may also exacerbate RLS.

Much of the evidence for pharmacological treatment in CC is extrapolated from patients with idiopathic restless legs. Gabapentin, dopamine agonists, co-careldopa and clonazepam are the treatments most commonly used, with varying results. All need dose reduction, and gabapentin in particular accumulates rapidly without dialysis and should be used with extreme caution in CC patients [21].

Sleep Disturbance

A detailed history of any sleep disturbance is important, in order to identify sleep apnoea, restless legs syndrome and pruritus, which may be underlying the problem and need treating, in their own right, initially. General sleep hygiene measures are important; avoiding caffeine after lunch, reducing overall caffeine intake, avoiding alcohol (which is both depressant and stimulant) and daytime sleeping. If sleep apnoea is excluded and other exacerbating symptoms treated optimally, and if general measures are unsuccessful, hypnotics may be necessary. Ideally they should be short term, and attempts to re-establish sleep patterns should be made. For those with a longer prognosis, hypnotics carry risk of dependence, and this needs consideration in CC management. The shorter-acting hypnotics, such as zolpidem 5–10 mg, or temazepam 7.5–10 mg are preferable. Longer-acting agents should be avoided as next day overhang sedation may increase the risk of falls.

Breathlessness

The most common causes of breathlessness or dyspnoea in the renal patient are anaemia and pulmonary oedema related to fluid overload or to coexisting cardio-vascular or respiratory disease. It is important to identify the cause since treating the cause is almost always the most appropriate and effective first line of management. Once treatment of the underlying cause has been exhausted, then symptomatic measures to relieve breathlessness will be required. These include general and non-pharmacological measures, psychological support and pharmacological measures.

General measures in advanced disease include sitting upright rather than lying (which maximises vital capacity), using a fan or stream of cool air that can provide effective symptom relief, inhaled oxygen if hypoxia is confirmed or suspected and a calm, settled environment. For the patient whose mobility is limited by breathlessness, physiotherapy and occupational therapy can help to maximise mobility and provide appropriate aids to improve function constrained by breathlessness. Since breathlessness is a profoundly unpleasant symptom, assessment and management of the underlying psychological state is important. Breathlessness is very commonly associated with anxiety, often in an escalating cycle (anxiety causing worsening dyspnoea, which triggers worsening anxiety, and so on). Information, education and support of patient and family are therefore critical.

As prognosis worsens, general and non-pharmacological measures will have less to offer, and pharmacological measures directed at the symptom of breathlessness itself may be more appropriate.

Pharmacological treatments directed specifically at breathlessness include low-dose opioids and benzodiazepines (especially if there is moderate or severe associated anxiety). However, there are considerable constraints on the use of opioids in renal patients; the guidance as for pain management should be followed, although dose of opioids for breathlessness is likely to be notably smaller (usually half or quarter the starting dose for pain) and titration upwards is usually not necessary. If small doses are not at least partly effective, combining an opioid such as fentanyl with low-dose midazolam towards the end of life (last few days or hours) may bring relief where either alone is only partially effective. This is often a better strategy than increasing the dose, since adverse effects quickly increase as doses rise.

Benzodiazepines are useful when there is coexisting anxiety but need to be used with care and in reduced doses. Shorter-acting benzodiazepines are recommended, such as lorazepam 0.5 mg orally or sublingually QID (if used sublingually, it has a quicker onset of action and may more readily restore a sense of control to the frightened and anxious patient). If the patient is in the last days of life, midazolam (at 25 % of normal dose if eGFR < 10) can be given subcutaneously and titrated according to effect. Midazolam can be given every 2–4 h, although ESRD patients are sensitive to its effects and do not usually need frequent or large doses. A starting dose of 1.25 or 2.5 mg is often sufficient. If more than one or two doses are required, a subcutaneous infusion over 24 h is most practical. Opiates may have a role as death approaches [22].

Conclusions

People with advanced renal disease who receive CC have extensive need for symptom control, psychological and social support as well as optimal disease management to minimise complications and maintain their residual renal function. They, therefore, need significant medical, nursing, psychological, spiritual and social care particularly as their illness advances towards end of life. High levels of coordination and collaboration between caregivers are paramount. Shared and appropriately informed decision-making backed up by effective and accessible care is recommended.

Key Points
- With increased longevity, advanced stage 5 chronic kidney disease (eGFR < 15 ml/min) has become an increasingly common problem, particularly in frail patients with multiple co-morbidities.
- Current evidence suggests that the survival advantage provided by dialysis is equivocal in patients who are over eighty years with multiple co-morbidities and have poor functional status.
- Initiation of dialysis is often associated with significant cognitive and functional decline in frail elderly patients.
- Over the past decade, a legitimate non-dialytic or conservative care (CC) option has emerged whereby emphasis is shifted towards preservation of residual renal function, symptom identification and management, attention to patient perceived priorities and de-medicalisation of death.
- Limited evidence suggests that quality of life is more favourable and that the number of out-of-hospital and intervention-free days is at least as many in CC patients. They are also less likely to die in acute hospital setting.
- Early and honest discussions about prognosis and patient-centred priorities are advised so that appropriate CC choices can be made and harm avoided.
- A new trajectory of functional decline is seen in CC patients that remains stable until shortly before death when a sharp and short-lived decline is observed.
- When a patient is unable to participate in a dialysis decision and dialysis is not expected to extend life significantly, CC is a reasonable alternative as evidence suggests that dialysis does not alleviate overall symptom burden.

References

1. Thorsteinsdottir B, Montori V, Prokop L, Murad MH (2013) Ageism vs the technical imperative, applying the GRADE framework to the evidence on haemodialysis in very elderly patients. Clin Interv Aging 8:797–807
2. Murtagh FE, Addington-Hall J, Higginson IJ (2007) The prevalence of symptoms in end-stage renal disease: a systematic review. Adv Chronic Kidney Dis 14(1):82–99

3. Jassal SV, Chiu E, Hladunewich M (2009) Loss of independence in patients starting dialysis at over 80 years of age or older. N Engl J Med 361(16):1612–1613
4. O'Connor N, Kmar P (2012) Conservative management of end-stage renal disease without dialysis: a systematic review. J Palliat Med 15(2):228–234
5. Schell J, Da Silva-Gane M, Germain M (2013) Recent insights into life expectancy with and without dialysis, vol 22(2). www.co-nephrolhypertens.com
6. Isaacs A, Burns A, Davenport A (2012) Should maximum conservative management be the standard paradigm for very elderly adults with chronic kidney disease or is there a role for dialysis? J Am Geriatr Soc 60(7):1376–1378
7. Carson RC, Juszczak M, Davenport A, Burns A (2009) Is maximum conservative management an equivalent treatment option to dialysis for elderly patients with significant comorbid disease? Clin J Am Soc Nephrol 4(10):1611–1619
8. Hussain JA, Mooney A, Russon L (2013) Comparison of survival analysis and palliative care involvement in patients aged over 70 years choosing conservative management or renal replacement therapy in advanced chronic kidney disease. Palliat Med 27:829–839
9. Da Silva-Gane M, Welisted D, Greenshields H, Norton S, Chandna SM, Farrington K (2012) Quality of life and survival in patients with advanced kidney failure managed conservatively or by dialysis. Clin J Am Soc Nephrol 7(12):2002–2009
10. Murtagh FE, Marsh JE, Donohoe P, Ekbal NJ, Sheerin NS, Harris FE (2007) Dialysis or not? A comparative survival study of patients over 75 years with chronic kidney disease stage 5. Nephrol Dial Transplant 22(7):1955–1962
11. Murtagh FE, Addington-Hall JM, Higginson IJ (2011) End-stage renal disease: a new trajectory of functional decline in the last year of life. J Am Geriatr Soc 59(2):304–308
12. Murtagh FEM, Chai MO, Donohoe P, Edmonds PM, Higginson IJ (2007) The use of opioid analgesia in end-stage renal disease patients managed without dialysis: recommendations for practice. J Pain Palliat Care Pharmacother 21(2):5–16
13. Goncalves AR, Ahmed AK, El Kossi M, El Nahas M (2011) Stopping rennin-angiotensin system inhibitors in chronic kidney disease: predictors of response. Nephron Clin Pract 119(4):348–354
14. Morton RL, Tong A, Howard K, Snelling P, Webster AC (2010) The views of patients and carers in treatment decision making for chronic kidney disease: systematic review an thematic synthesis of qualitative studies. BMJ 340:c112
15. Morton RL, Snelling P, Webster AC et al (2012) Factors influencing patient choice of dialysis versus conservative care to treat end-stage kidney disease. CMAJ 184(5):E277–E283
16. Van De Luijtgaarden MW, Noordzij M et al (2013) Conservative care in Europe- nephrologists' experience with the decision not to start renal replacement therapy. Nephrol Dial Transplant 28:2604–2612
17. Davison SN, Torgunrud C (2007) The creation of an advance care planning process for patients with ESRD. Am J Kidney Dis 49(1):27–36
18. NHS Kidney Care GMMKC, Advanced Renal Care (ARC) Project (2012) Getting it right: end of life care in advanced kidney disease
19. Lee BO, Lin CC, Chaboyer W, Chiang CL, Hung CC (2007) The fatigue experience of haemodialysis patients in Taiwan. J Clin Nurs 16(2):407–413
20. Keithi-Reddy SR, Patel TV, Armstrong AW, Singh AK (2007) Uremic pruritus. Kidney Int 72(3):373–377
21. Medcalf P, Bhatia KP (2006) Restless legs syndrome. BMJ 333(7566):457–458
22. Jennings AL, Davies AN, Higgins JP, Gibbs JS, Broadley KE (2002) A systematic review of the use of opioids in the management of dyspnoea. Thorax 57(11):939–944

Chapter 15
Unplanned Start of Hemodialysis and Transition to Community

Preethi Yerram

Introduction

Advances in medicine have helped fight disease allowing people to live longer, albeit with a myriad of chronic medical conditions. There is no universally accepted definition of "elderly, old, or older" person, but the generally accepted age range for this cohort is over 65 years. Those over the age of 80 years are considered "very-elderly."

There has been a surge in the number of older patients with end-stage renal disease starting dialysis therapies in the recent years. According to the recent 2012 USRDS report, patients in the 75 years and older age group was the fastest growing cohort of ESRD patients followed by those between 65 and 74 years of age [1]. Elderly dialysis patients also have poor survival – a mean survival of 24.9 months in those between 65 and 79 years, progressively decreasing with increasing age, to 8.4 months in those over 90 [2].

The USRDS data is also very revealing in that the majority of ESRD patients are not receiving optimal pre-ESRD care. This results in a disproportionate number of patients starting hemodialysis (HD) with a catheter [1].

There is limited published literature pertaining to unplanned dialysis initiation and its outcomes, and only a handful of publications are specific to the elderly population. As a result, general observations made from these studies are often extrapolated to the elderly patient cohort.

P. Yerram, MD, MS, FASN
Division of Nephrology and Hypertension, Department of Medicine,
University of Missouri-Columbia School of Medicine, 1 Hospital
Dr CSE Building, Room CE 417, Columbia, MO, 65212, USA
e-mail: yerramp@health.misouri.edu

© Springer Science+Business Media New York 2016
M. Misra (ed.), *Dialysis in Older Adults: A Clinical Handbook*,
DOI 10.1007/978-1-4939-3320-4_15

What Is "Unplanned Start" of Dialysis? Defining the Terminology

Review of literature suggests that there has been much variability in the definition of "unplanned dialysis." In general, dialysis is considered "planned," when it is initiated in a scheduled, outpatient setting with the use of a permanent vascular or peritoneal access. On the other hand, any unscheduled initiation of dialysis with or without the use of a permanent access is considered "unplanned." Most patients initiating dialysis in an unplanned setting are started on HD with a central venous catheter (CVC), as it is the "path of least resistance."

The lack of consistency and uniformity in the terminology and definition of "unplanned dialysis" can make data gathering across studies challenging, which in turn makes deduction of outcomes difficult and unreliable. As a result, an alternative term, "suboptimal initiation" was proposed to define this better and recommended including those patients that initiate dialysis (a) in the hospital or (b) with a central venous catheter or (c) not on the chronic dialysis modality of their choice. Creating a broader awareness for the consistent use of this term is recommended to help with standardization and for research purposes.

The rate of suboptimal dialysis initiation has ranged from 24 to 49 % in different studies [3] and has been noted to be a problem in patients with and without pre-ESRD nephrology care.

Causes of Suboptimal Dialysis Initiation

Several reasons have been cited in the literature as being responsible for suboptimal dialysis initiation, including late referral to nephrology (defined as nephrology care <1 year prior to initiation of dialysis) or difficulties in accessing nephrology care due to insurance or financial reasons, acute or chronic kidney disease, patient-related issues such as being in denial/refusing referral to education for RRT, and lack of proper surgical resources for establishment of a permanent dialysis access (Table 15.1).

Table 15.1 Causes of suboptimal initiation of dialysis

1. Late referral to nephrology/difficulty accessing nephrology/specialty care due to insurance or financial reasons
2. Acute on chronic kidney disease
3. Patient-related issues such as being in denial/refusing referral for education and preparation for RRT
4. Lack of proper surgical resources for establishment of a permanent dialysis access, such as difficulty with referral, insufficient surgical expertise

While one may assume that early referral to nephrology would prevent suboptimal dialysis initiation, data suggest otherwise [1].

Suboptimal dialysis initiation is a significant problem in patients with and without pre-ESRD nephrology care with the majority of incident ESRD patients starting dialysis "suboptimally," utilizing a central venous catheter (CVC). Furthermore, these patients were noted to have a higher mortality rate in the first 6 months of dialysis initiation, and any benefit conferred by early nephrology referral was vitiated by suboptimal dialysis initiation [4].

Studies investigating the factors associated with suboptimal initiation in patients referred to nephrology prior to their dialysis start found that acute on chronic kidney disease, patient-related delays, delays attributed to renal service (relating to timely referral for modality education, access creation), and surgical delays were some of the common causes of suboptimal dialysis initiation (Table 15.2) [5, 6]. Also, the risk of suboptimal initiation increased by 4 % with each one-year increment in age [5].

Outcomes of Suboptimal Dialysis Initiation

Suboptimal dialysis initiation has been associated with poor outcomes with increased morbidity and mortality, higher rates of hospitalization/associated costs with increased economic burden to the healthcare system, increased use of CVCs (associated with higher rates of infection and attendant complications), and a negative impact on the patients' ability to choose a modality of their choice (Table 15.3).

Table 15.2 Causes of suboptimal initiation in patients with pre-ESRD nephrology care >12 months

1. Patient-related
2. Acute on chronic kidney disease
3. Surgical delays
4. Late decision-making by the nephrologist

Table 15.3 Outcomes of suboptimal dialysis initiation

1. Higher mortality
2. Higher rates of hospitalization, blood transfusions
3. Worse metabolic profile
4. Higher costs to healthcare system
5. Lower quality of life
6. Increased use of central venous catheters and higher rate of infections
7. Inability to initiate with dialysis modality of choice

Mortality and Hospitalization Outcomes

Unplanned start leads to an increased risk of mortality as well as higher rates of blood transfusion and subsequent hospitalization, when compared to those that started electively [4, 7–10]. For patients over 75 years of age, late referral and unprepared access were noted to confer higher mortality risk than mortality related to 5-year age increments [8].

Economic Outcomes

Suboptimal dialysis initiation is also associated with increased economic burden, with studies noting severalfold increased per-patient cost for suboptimal initiation compared to optimal initiation. This was mainly attributed to the need for hospitalization and the need for higher number of in-hospital dialysis sessions [9, 11].

Quality of Life Outcomes

The manner of dialysis initiation may have a bearing on the quality of life (QoL). Planned dialysis initiation may be associated with better QoL independent of comorbidities, suggesting that the QoL benefit may not be due to selection bias [12]. Similar findings were noted in another study involving elderly incident ESRD patients (>70 years old). Those with suboptimal dialysis initiation had a lower QoL, higher rate of pulmonary and peripheral edema, digestive disorders, and anorexia, as well as significantly lower levels of sodium and hematocrit compared to those with optimal initiation. Futhermore, QoL in ESRD patients undergoing optimal dialysis initiation was similar to controls without chronic kidney disease [13].

Strategies to Prevent Suboptimal Initiation

Prevention of suboptimal dialysis initiation entails addressing and resolving the underlying factors that are responsible for this problem. Late referral to a nephrologist is one of the factors associated with suboptimal initiation as previously discussed, and this has been associated with poor outcomes. This problem can be addressed by increasing awareness and educating the primary care providers (PCPs) about the adverse socioeconomic, mortality/morbidity, and QOL outcomes associated with late referral and suboptimal initiation. Providing information and tools to primary care providers to identify patients with kidney disease who are potentially headed towards dialysis can decrease the number of late referrals This is very important as PCPs are usually the first line of contact for patients with kidney disease. A timely referral by the PCPs will allow for provision of effective pre-dialysis education, so that the patient can make an informed choice about the modality, plan for it accordingly, and avoid suboptimal dialysis initiation.

The advent of chronic kidney disease (CKD) guidelines by work groups such as KDOQI (Kidney Disease Outcomes Quality Initiative) and KDIGO (Kidney Disease Improving Global Outcomes) [14] has improved awareness regarding the criteria for referral to a nephrologist. Nephrology referral is warranted when the estimated glomerular filtration rate (eGFR) drops below 30 ml/min or in cases of rapid progression of CKD (decline in eGFR of more than 5 ml/min/1.73 m²/year). Once a patient is referred to the nephrologist, a multidisciplinary team care approach (involving the nephrologist, dietitian, social worker, pharmacist, and a CKD educator with a thorough knowledge of management of CKD-ESRD and its complications) seems to lead to improved overall patient care.

Dialysis education is usually recommended at an eGFR of <30 ml/min, followed by a decision concerning modality between 20 and 30 ml/min.

Pre-dialysis education can determine whether dialysis initiation would be planned or unplanned. The beneficial effect of multidisciplinary care (MDC) in providing pre-dialysis education has been shown in a few studies. Care in the setting of an MDC clinic along with standard nephrology care is known to be associated with a better metabolic profile (higher hemoglobin, albumin, calcium) and lower morbidity and mortality [15]. Patients with multidisciplinary pre-dialysis care are also more likely to have a functioning access at the time of dialysis initiation, fewer hospitalizations, and deaths at 1 year. Lack of MDC and older age and cardiovascular disease are known to be independently associated with increased mortality on dialysis [16].

Transition to the Community

Without further education, most patients with suboptimal hemodialysis start tend to choose in-center HD as their permanent dialysis modality of choice [17]. This may especially be true in case of the elderly patients, as they are often perceived as being "unsuitable" for a home dialysis therapy possibly due to concerns regarding their frailty, physical and cognitive functioning, and lack of social support. However, with proper education (Fig. 15.1) and understanding of the patient's support systems and possible barriers to pursuing a home therapy, we may be able to offer alternatives (such as assisted PD) and provide the needed support for patients to pursue home dialysis if they should so desire.

As previously discussed, increased mortality and frailty for elderly dialysis patients has been well documented. These issues need to be factored into the discussion and education provided to patients and their caregivers. Depending on the patient's overall condition and other prevalent comorbidities, it may be appropriate to discuss conservative management/hospice care in lieu of continuing dialysis.

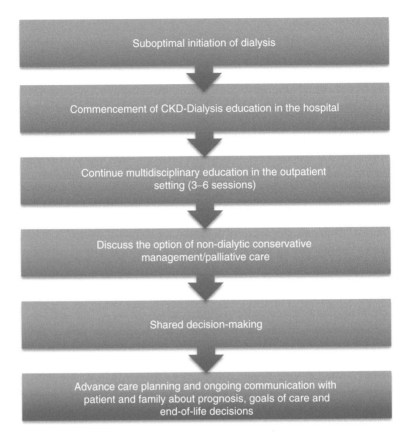

Fig. 15.1 Algorithm for transition after suboptimal initiation

An in-hospital CKD-education program for patients with suboptimal dialysis initiation has been shown to increase the number of patients choosing a home dialysis modality for maintenance (35 %) compared to the rates prior to the implementation of the in-hospital education program (13 %) [17]. Also, education of suboptimal HD patients by a renal triage nurse (RTN) may also help achieve similar results [18]. These data suggest that patients with suboptimal dialysis start will benefit from a CKD-education program that is initiated in the hospital and continued as an outpatient, and efforts should be made to facilitate this.

For CKD-dialysis patients to have a good understanding of their disease process, prognosis, pros and cons of different dialysis modalities, generally, 3–6 educational sessions are recommended [19], and these should include information pertaining to non-dialytic conservative management and possibly palliative/hospice care if appropriate.

The concept of advance care planning (ACP) is also gaining ground, which includes ongoing communication between patients, their families, and health care providers about the patients' wishes regarding their end-of-life care. ACP calls for continuing discussion about the prognosis, goals of care, and patient's preferences as the patient's health deteriorates and end-of-life issues become more relevant [20]. ACP also facilitates change in ESRD therapy if patient desires, as patients can change their mind with ongoing education and communication. Having advance care directives and a healthcare proxy in place is part of ACP [21]. Such patients use less invasive procedures and pursue hospice care sooner, and more frequently [22].

In summary, a smooth transition to the community after suboptimal dialysis initiation requires multidisciplinary CKD-dialysis education that starts in the hospital and continues as an outpatient until the patient is able to make an informed decision, after weighing in all his options.

Conclusion

There is an increase in the number of elderly patients starting dialysis, and a significant proportion of these patients initiate dialysis suboptimally. Suboptimal dialysis initiation is associated with adverse mortality, hospitalization, economic, and QoL outcomes. Several factors are responsible for suboptimal initiation including late referral to the nephrologist, patient-related factors, lack of surgical resources, and delay in decision-making on part of the nephrologists. Prevention of suboptimal dialysis starts requires a concerted effort to address the underlying factors that lead to this problem in the first place. Educating and aiding the PCPs to identify CKD patients that are likely to progress to ESRD and referring them early to a nephrologist is vital to avoiding late referrals. In addition, multidisciplinary CKD-dialysis education is an important component of pre-dialysis care, which can improve outcomes and increase the likelihood of optimal dialysis initiation. Given the significant burden and increased mortality with dialysis in the elderly, the options of non-dialytic conservative management, time-limited trial of dialysis, and palliative/hospice care should be included in the patient-education program. Advance care planning and ongoing communication with patients and their families will allow a smooth transition when end-of-life care decisions need to be made.

Key Points
1. Unplanned or suboptimal dialysis initiation is a major problem in the elderly ESRD patients.
2. Suboptimal dialysis initiation is associated with adverse mortality, hospitalization, economic, and QoL outcomes.
3. Multidisciplinary patient education is vital in countering the problem of suboptimal initiation as it helps patients make an informed choice and start dialysis in an optimal manner.
4 Shared decision making and advance care planning are important strategies to maintain an ongoing communication with patients and their families about goals of care and end-of-life decisions when appropriate.

References

1. U S Renal Data System (2012) USRDS 2012 annual data report: atlas of chronic kidney disease and end-stage renal disease in the United States. National Institutes of Health, National Institute of Diabetes and Digestive and Kidney Diseases, Bethesda
2. Kurella M et al (2007) Octogenarians and nonagenarians starting dialysis in the United States. Ann Intern Med 146(3):177–183
3. Mendelssohn DC, Malmberg C, Hamandi B (2009) An integrated review of "unplanned" dialysis initiation: reframing the terminology to "suboptimal" initiation. BMC Nephrol 10:22
4. Mendelssohn DC et al (2011) Suboptimal initiation of dialysis with and without early referral to a nephrologist. Nephrol Dial Transplant 26(9):2959–2965
5. Buck J et al (2007) Why do patients known to renal services still undergo urgent dialysis initiation? A cross-sectional survey. Nephrol Dial Transplant 22(11):3240–3245
6. Hughes SA et al (2013) Factors associated with suboptimal initiation of dialysis despite early nephrologist referral. Nephrol Dial Transplant 28(2):392–397
7. Metcalfe W et al (2000) Can we improve early mortality in patients receiving renal replacement therapy? Kidney Int 57(6):2539–2545
8. Foote C et al (2012) Survival of elderly dialysis patients is predicted by both patient and practice characteristics. Nephrol Dial Transplant 27(9):3581–3587
9. Gorriz JL et al (2002) Prognostic significance of programmed dialysis in patients who initiate renal substitutive treatment. Multicenter study in Spain. Nefrologia 22(1):49–59
10. Couchoud C et al (2007) Associations between comorbidities, treatment choice and outcome in the elderly with end-stage renal disease. Nephrol Dial Transplant 22(11):3246–3254
11. Information, C.I.f.H (2008) The cost of hospital stays: why costs vary. CIHI, Ottawa
12. Caskey FJ et al (2003) Early referral and planned initiation of dialysis: what impact on quality of life? Nephrol Dial Transplant 18(7):1330–1338
13. Loos C et al (2003) Effect of end-stage renal disease on the quality of life of older patients. J Am Geriatr Soc 51(2):229–233
14. Group., K.D.I.G.O.K.C.W (2013) KDIGO 2012 clinical practice guideline for the evaluation and management of chronic kidney disease. Kidney Int Suppl 3(1):1–150
15. Curtis BM et al (2005) The short- and long-term impact of multi-disciplinary clinics in addition to standard nephrology care on patient outcomes. Nephrol Dial Transplant 20(1):147–154
16. Goldstein M et al (2004) Multidisciplinary predialysis care and morbidity and mortality of patients on dialysis. Am J Kidney Dis 44(4):706–714
17. Rioux JP et al (2011) Effect of an in-hospital chronic kidney disease education program among patients with unplanned urgent-start dialysis. Clin J Am Soc Nephrol 6(4):799–804
18. Hanko J et al (2011) Dedication of a nurse to educating suboptimal haemodialysis starts improved transition to independent modalities of renal replacement therapy. Nephrol Dial Transplant 26(7):2302–2308
19. Saggi SJ et al (2012) Considerations in the optimal preparation of patients for dialysis. Nat Rev Nephrol 8(7):381–389
20. Davison SN (2006) Facilitating advance care planning for patients with end-stage renal disease: the patient perspective. Clin J Am Soc Nephrol 1(5):1023–1028
21. Holley JL (2005) Palliative care in end-stage renal disease: focus on advance care planning, hospice referral, and bereavement. Semin Dial 18(2):154–156
22. Kurella Tamura M, Cohen LM (2010) Should there be an expanded role for palliative care in end-stage renal disease? Curr Opin Nephrol Hypertens 19(6):556–560

Chapter 16
Shared Decision-Making: Role of the Nephrologist in Palliative Care

Robert G. Fassett

It is imperative that the nephrologist focuses on an assessment of the patient's symptoms and is fully cognizant of the therapies that are indicated in palliative care of patients with ESRD. These differ significantly from those used in the general population as side effects of commonly used drugs can be distressing to patients with ESRD.

Introduction

With the increasing presentation and acceptance of the elderly, often with multiple comorbidities, onto ESRD programs, there has been heightened awareness of the need to address palliative care issues not only for those on dialysis but also prior to the onset of ESRD and the need for ESRD therapy [1].

The World Health Organization (WHO) defines palliative care as "the active total care of patients whose disease is not responsive to curative treatment and includes control of pain, other symptoms, together with attention to psychological, social, and spiritual problems." The WHO definition further asserts that *palliative care should not be limited to patients at the end of life*. Rather, it is designed to improve the quality of life (QOL) of all patients suffering from chronic, life-limiting illness regardless of life expectancy.

Advanced care planning is an integral component of palliative care and includes the ethical, psychological, and spiritual issues related to starting, continuing, withholding, and stopping dialysis. It is the process of clarifying preferences and individual plans for care near the end of life. The advanced care plan needs to be patient

R.G. Fassett, BMedSc, MBBS, PhD, FRACP, FASN
School of Human Movement Studies and Nutritional Sciences, The University of Queensland, Rm 535 Connell Building St Lucia, 4072 Brisbane, QC, Australia
e-mail: r.fassett@uq.edu.au

© Springer Science+Business Media New York 2016
M. Misra (ed.), *Dialysis in Older Adults: A Clinical Handbook*,
DOI 10.1007/978-1-4939-3320-4_16

specific and periodic updating is required. Ultimately when the patient is dying and the advanced care plan needs to be considered, their recorded preferences should be respected.

The nephrologists' desired outcomes from advanced care planning include an enhanced understanding by the patient and their family of the trajectory of their disease and hence prognosis, along with their end-of-life issues. This allows greater patient autonomy and satisfaction for the patient and their family. It assists the patient in finding hope, a meaning to life, and spiritual settlement along with strengthened relationships with their loved ones.

Advanced care directives include the living wills and durable powers of attorney for healthcare and are the legal documents which vary across jurisdictions. This is only one component of advanced care planning.

Withdrawal of dialysis is one of the commonest causes of death among dialysis patients. Hence, the nephrologist must prepare the patient for this possibility well in advance and be experienced and sensitive to when this needs to be considered.

Palliative Care in Patients with ESRD

The timely involvement of the palliative care team in the management of the patient with ESRD is important. The point during the patient's illness that this occurs will depend on the individual patient and the experience and training of the nephrologist. In other disease states such as non-small cell lung cancer, early involvement of palliative care has even improved survival [2]. Multidisciplinary management of stage 4–5 CKD patients with a focus on advanced care planning and directives will ensure patients make the best decisions for their future. These plans must be continually reviewed as circumstances change during the trajectory of their illness.

The nephrologist plays the central role within the multidisciplinary team as the patient's physician. The other key healthcare providers include renal nurses, social workers, psychologists, palliative care clinicians, dietitians, and spiritual supporters.

Davison et al. surveyed and assessed the nephrologist's preparedness for decisions at the end of life [3]. This survey was conducted in 2005 and contemporary practice may have changed. However, 39 % of nephrologists perceived they were well prepared to make end-of-life decisions. However, of concern, this suggests 61 % were not. An awareness of decision-making guidelines, experience with making dialysis withdrawal decisions, and nephrologist age >46 years were associated with greater perceived preparedness. This suggests the contemporary nephrologist would be best placed to make end-of-life decisions if they familiarize themselves with the many available guidelines relevant to this area.

The discussions surrounding the pathway a patient takes should be initiated early; preferably in CKD stage 4 when eGFR reaches around 25 ml/min/1.73 m^2. This of course depends on the rate of decline of eGFR as well. If the eGFR is very stable, then discussions may be premature, but if the eGFR is rapidly declining, discussions may need to occur earlier. Once the nephrologist recognizes the trigger point, the discussion of the following issues should be lead by the nephrologist.

For those patients with ESRD on dialysis, the trigger to discuss dialysis withdrawal is often the occurrence of a significant comorbid event such as a stroke or the development of a malignancy. Sometimes it is simply the patient's request once their QOL declines.

The Role of the Nephrologist

1. The nephrologist should take the lead role in the discussions around palliative care as with all aspects of the patient's management. The discussions will cover the options for therapy including choosing a non-dialysis pathway supported by palliative care or alternatively progressing to dialysis. Specifically, the nephrologist should initiate this with the patient at a clinical consultation. Subsequently, the nephrologist should organize consultations involving the family and the other members of the multidisciplinary team with the consent of the patient. An ongoing dialogue at subsequent consultations will be necessary to reinforce material discussed as patients often forget or misinterpret information at initial discussions. It is the responsibility of the nephrologist to ensure the patient receives consistent information from all members of the multidisciplinary team. This is to avoid confusing the patient at such a sensitive time.

    Based on a survey conducted by Davison, 51.9 % of dialysis patients had not had any discussion of end-of-life care in the 12-months preceding the survey and only 9.9 % had such a discussion with their nephrologist. The survey showed 60.7 % of patient's regretted starting dialysis and only 34.2 % started dialysis because of their own specific wish; the rest started because of the wishes of their family or doctor [4]. For most patients (90.4 %), the nephrologist had not talked to them about how long they had left to live.

2. The nephrologist should discuss the best estimate of the patients' likely survival should they select to have dialysis. Recent studies have made this aspect a little easier [5, 6]. For example, if the patient is over 75 years of age with multiple comorbidities, one can reasonably indicate that the patients' survival will be not significantly better if they chose dialysis [5]. Also, if the patient is a nursing home resident in the USA, one can estimate that functional capacity is unlikely to be retained at 12 months (in 13 % only) after initiation of dialysis and that 58 % of patients will have died [6]. The nephrologist may choose one or several of the predictive tools summarized below to assist this estimation.

3. The nephrologist should discuss the QOL the patient is likely to experience should they select to have dialysis treatment. Results from a survey conducted in dialysis patients by Davison found 57.2 % felt relief of pain or discomfort and improved quality of life was preferable to extending life [6].

4. The nephrologist should ensure there is an accurate compassionate assessment of the patient's symptoms. Any symptoms should be treated according to specific renal guidelines. The nephrologist will be faced with many patients with multiple comorbidities, functional decline, psychological distress, and social challenges. Ameliorating symptoms will improve QOL and allay anxiety.

5. The nephrologist must ensure that the elderly dialysis patient is not subjected to unnecessary life prolongation and distress. The United States Renal Data System (USRDS) and Medicare data 2004–2009 revealed that 80 % of dialysis patients had a dialysis procedure performed within 30 days of their death and were hospitalized for twice as many days as terminal cancer patients. Thus, the nephrologist should take overall responsibility in such situations and provide direction and leadership by facilitating the advanced care planning. These patients are often impeded by cognitive decline, which impairs the capacity to make decisions.

6. The nephrologist should use available clinical prediction models to assist decisions about starting or withdrawal of dialysis. These are summarized below.

Clinical Prediction Models

The nephrologist can use several prediction models to assist in estimation of the prognosis of elderly patients with ESKD. These are summarized in Table 16.1. A simple method is the validated "surprise question" which asks, "Would you be surprised if the patient died in the next year?" This is by far the easiest method as it can be done at the bedside. The other scores require additional information such as the tool developed by Couchoud, which incorporates clinical parameters and gives an estimated 6-month mortality risk of between 8 and 70 % (Table 16.2). Another tool

Table 16.1 Prediction Models to estimate prognosis in elderly with ESKD

Clinical prediction models
The surprise question
The modified Charlson score (MCS)
The JAMA Kidney Failure Risk Equation
Combination of MCS and surprise question
Couchoud 6-month prognosis score

Risk factors	Points
Total dependence for transfers	3
BMI <18.5 kg/m^2	2
Peripheral vascular disease stage 3 or 4	2
Congestive heart failure stage 3 or 4	2
Severe behavioral disorder	2
Unplanned dialysis initiation	2
Active malignancy	1
Diabetes mellitus	1
Dysrhythmia	1

Total score	6-months mortality rate
0	8 %
1	8–10 %
2	14–17 %
3–4	21–26 %
5–6	33–35 %
7–8	50–51 %
≥9	62–70 %

Table 16.2 Couchoud prognosis score for prognosis in the elderly with ESRD [7]

Table 16.3 Modified
Charlson comorbidity score
for prognosis in the elderly
with ESRD

Comorbidity	Score
Cancer	5
Myocardial infarct	2
Congestive cardiac failure	2
Cerebrovascular disease	2
Diabetes with complications	2
Liver disease	2
Peripheral vascular disease	1
Dementia	1
Chronic pulmonary disease	1
Rheumatologic disease	1
Peptic ulcer disease	1
Diabetes without complications	1

Table 16.4 Modified Charlson
score for prediction of survival

MCS	Predicted survival time (months)
9–15	<3
6–8	3–12
4–5	12–24
2–3	24–60
0–1	>60

designed by Cohen uses both the surprise question and four additional parameters: the presence or absence of dementia and peripheral vascular disease, age, and serum albumin. This tool can be accessed using an app available online at www.qxmd.com/apps/calculate-by-qxmd.

Another such tool is the modified Charlson score (MCS) is adapted from the Charlson Comorbidity index and identifies dialysis patients likely to have a 1-year mortality rate of 50 %. The score is derived from the sum of the patient's comorbidities (Table 16.3) and their age. The age score is based on one point per decade from the age of 40 years. This gives a predicted survival time in months (Table 16.4).

Finally, the JAMA Kidney Failure Risk Equation uses laboratory test results and patient demographics to estimate the risk of progression to ESKD and the calculator is available as an app from www.qxmd.com/Kidney-Failure-Risk-Equation.

The Renal Physicians Association has also produced guidelines to help the nephrologist and the patients and families make the difficult decisions regarding starting and withdrawing from dialysis. The recommendations for establishing a shared decision-making relationship are outlined in Table 16.5.

The physical and psychological symptom burden that stage 5 ESRD patients have during the last month of their life can be greater or similar to that of terminal cancer patients. The Liverpool Care Pathway through guidelines outlines the best available evidence for providing therapy for treatment of patients dying from ESRD. A United Kingdom Expert Consensus Group also developed evidence-based

Table 16.5 Summarized Renal Physician Association guidelines

1. Establish a physician-patient relationship for shared decision-making
2. Fully inform ESKD patients of their diagnosis, prognosis, treatment options
3. Give all patients a prognosis specific to their overall condition
4. Institute advanced care planning and an advanced care directive
5. Withhold initiating or withdraw dialysis in clearly defined circumstances[a]   Fully informed patients with capacity who refuse dialysis or request its withdrawal   Patients without capacity with an advanced directive   Patients without capacity whose legal guardian refuse dialysis or request its withdrawal   Patients with irreversible profound neurological impairment
6. Forgo dialysis when prognosis is very poor or if it cannot be performed safely   Patients whose condition makes it technically impossible to provide dialysis   Presence of a nonrenal terminal illness such as cancer   Age >75, "no" to surprise question, high comorbidity score, poor functional capacity, or malnutrition
7. Consider time-limited dialysis trial if prognosis uncertain and no consensus
8. Establish conflict resolution process for dialysis decision disagreement
9. Offer palliative care services to all ESKD patients with disease burden
10. Use systematic approach to communicate diagnosis, prognosis, and treatment options and goals of care

[a]Palliative care is an integral part of the medical management with a focus on symptom relief, comfort, and QOL. This is led by the nephrologist with input from the multidisciplinary palliative care team

Table 16.6 Symptom control in the dying patient with ESKD, summarized from the United Kingdom Expert Consensus Group [8]

Symptom	Treatment recommendations
Nausea and vomiting	Haloperidol (half usual dose)
	Levomepromazine (alternative)
	Metoclopramide (avoid greater risk of extrapyramidal reaction)
	Cyclizine (avoid hypotension and tachyarrhythmia)
Respiratory secretions	Glycopyrronium (half dose)
	Hyoscine butylbromide (alternative)
	Hyoscine hydrobromide (avoid, drowsiness, agitation)
Terminal agitation	Midazolam at reduced dose and increased dose interval
	Levomepromazine (alternative)
Pain and/or dyspnea	Fentanyl (subcutaneous)
	Alfentanil (alternative) (continuous infusion)
	Oxycodone, hydromorphone, diamorphine (short term if alternatives unavailable)
	Morphine, diamorphine (avoid regular or continuous infusion)

guidelines for symptom control in patients dying from ESKD [8]. The recommendations are summarized in Table 16.6.

Figure 16.1 outlines our understanding of management of CKD over time. It arbitrarily divides overall management into: (i) the technical issues related to the kidney disease and its comorbidities and their treatment, (ii) the immediate symp-

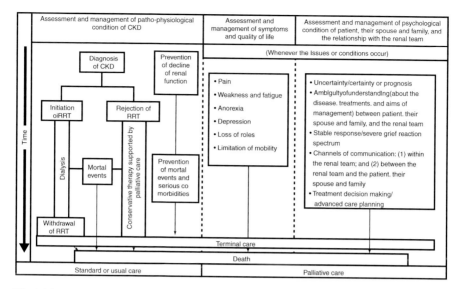

Fig. 16.1 An idealized model of care for patients with ESKD incorporating palliative care [1]

toms and quality-of-life issues suffered by the patient, and (iii) psychological impact of the disease and its prognosis on the patient, their spouse and family, and how this affects communication and decision-making between them and the renal multidisciplinary team. Optimal patient care through the course of the disease will involve combining technically proficient disease assessment and management, attention to the immediate condition as perceived by the patient, and guidance of the emotional condition of the patient, their knowledge and understanding of their disease and its prognosis, in order to allow decision-making that maximally satisfies the patient and their family. The relationships between the components of care have not been made explicit, and the effects of symptomatic and psychological management, and quality of communication, on patient satisfaction have not been measured to any useful extent. The following category of patients might have difficulty in being brought into an effective partnership with their physicians in deciding on the nature and timing of transitions in their renal replacement therapy:

- Those who are uncertain about his/her prognosis
- Whose understanding differs significantly from their professional advisors
- Those suffering from denial or depression as a reaction to realizing their mortally threatening and severely restrictive disease
- Whose communication with the renal team seems to be at cross-purposes

However, evidence would be more helpful than speculation. The "standard or usual" and "palliative" designations do not imply separate functions, but might be regarded as integrated components of overall patient care. Current best practice will be intuitively performing these functions but is stated explicitly here to assist service planning and information recording and communication between the patient's healthcare providers. The list of activities is not intended to be exhaustive, but only illustrative of types of activity. Also, health-funding models, notably item-of-service payment, may need to be modified to facilitate this integrated model of care.

Although the nephrologist should lead discussions with the patient and their family, they should function in close collaboration with the multidisciplinary team. The varied skills of the renal nurses, social workers, psychologists, and palliative care professionals should be incorporated into the patients' care at levels dependent on the individual situation. The strengths of these professionals will vary individually and by institution. Thus, the nephrologist must lead this group in the context of palliative care for the patient with ESRD.

Conclusions

The nephrologist is the clinical leader and coordinates all aspects of palliative care for the patient with ESRD. They must be trained and familiar with the available contemporary guidelines appropriate to their practice location. Skills working as part of a multidisciplinary team are essential.

Key Points
1. Advanced care planning and directives.
   Nephrologists must ensure patients approaching end-stage renal disease (ESRD) and those established on dialysis have participated in advanced care planning and record an advanced care directive appropriate for the jurisdiction where they undertake their medical care. This must be regularly reviewed and supported by an accessible, recorded update. It is especially important to review and update the record when there are significant changes in the patient's clinical condition.
2. End-of-life decisions.
   End-of-life decisions at critical times in a patient's care trajectory will be significantly aided by prior advanced care planning and the availability of an advanced care directive. However, at these times, the nephrologist should lead the discussion around the end-of-life decisions with the patient and their family.
3. Palliative care.
   Depending on the resources available in the healthcare facility, the nephrologist may be the de facto palliative care provider or when available enlist a qualified palliative care physician in the management of the patient. Palliative care has increasingly been considered at earlier stages of life-limiting disease and according to the World Health Organization definition should be part of all such chronic disease care.

4. Withdrawal of therapy.
   Even with the creation of the best plans, patients who start dialysis are often faced with deteriorating health where quality of life is so poor that withdrawal of therapy is considered. The nephrologist must lead discussions with the patient and their family about all aspects of dialysis withdrawal.
5. Symptom assessment and treatment.

References

1. Fassett RG, Robertson IK, Mace R, Youl L, Challenor S, Bull R (2011) Palliative care in end-stage kidney disease. Nephrology (Carlton) 16(1):4–12
2. Temel JS, Greer JA, Muzikansky A et al (2010) Early palliative care for patients with metastatic non-small-cell lung cancer. N Engl J Med 363(8):733–742
3. Davison SN, Jhangri GS, Holley JL, Moss AH (2006) Nephrologists' reported preparedness for end-of-life decision-making. Clin J Am Soc Nephrol 1(6):1256–1262
4. Davison SN (2010) End-of-life care preferences and needs: perceptions of patients with chronic kidney disease. Clin J Am Soc Nephrol 5(2):195–204
5. Murtagh FE, Marsh JE, Donohoe P, Ekbal NJ, Sheerin NS, Harris FE (2007) Dialysis or not? A comparative survival study of patients over 75 years with chronic kidney disease stage 5. Nephrol Dial Transplant 22(7):1955–1962
6. Kurella Tamura M, Covinsky KE, Chertow GM, Yaffe K, Landefeld CS, McCulloch CE (2009) Functional status of elderly adults before and after initiation of dialysis. N Engl J Med 361(16):1539–1547
7. Couchoud C, Labeeuw M, Moranne O et al (2009) A clinical score to predict 6-month prognosis in elderly patients starting dialysis for end-stage renal disease. Nephrol Dial Transplant 24(5):1553–1561
8. Douglas C, Murtagh FE, Chambers EJ, Howse M, Ellershaw J (2009) Symptom management for the adult patient dying with advanced chronic kidney disease: a review of the literature and development of evidence-based guidelines by a United Kingdom Expert Consensus Group. Palliat Med 23(2):103–110

Erratum to: Anemia Management in the Elderly Dialysis Patient: Is It Different?

Iain C. Macdougall

Erratum to:
Chapter 9 in: Madhukar Misra, *Dialysis in Older Adults,*
DOI 10.1007/978-1-4939-3320-4_9

The labels were spelled incorrectly in Figure 9.2. The below revised image has been replaced with the corrected labels:

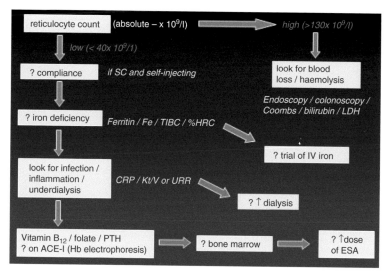

The online version of the original chapter can be found under
DOI:10.1007/978-1-4939-3320-4_9

I.C. Macdougall, BSc, MD, FRCP
Department of Renal Medicine, King's College Hospital, London, UK

Renal Unit, King's College Hospital, London SE5 9RS, UK
e-mail: iain.macdougall@nhs.net

© Springer Science+Business Media New York 2016
M. Misra (ed.), *Dialysis in Older Adults: A Clinical Handbook,*
DOI 10.1007/978-1-4939-3320-4_17

Index

© Springer Science+Business Media New York 2016
M. Misra (ed.), *Dialysis in Older Adults: A Clinical Handbook*,
DOI 10.1007/978-1-4939-3320-4

Printed in the United States
By Bookmasters